Natural Product from the Deep Sea

Natural Product from the Deep Sea

Editor

Kazuo Umezawa

MDPI • Basel • Beijing • Wuhan • Barcelona • Belgrade • Manchester • Tokyo • Cluj • Tianjin

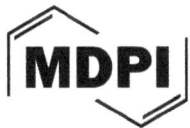

Editor
Kazuo Umezawa
Aichi Medical University
Japan

Editorial Office
MDPI
St. Alban-Anlage 66
4052 Basel, Switzerland

This is a reprint of articles from the Special Issue published online in the open access journal *Marine Drugs* (ISSN 1660-3397) (available at: https://www.mdpi.com/journal/marinedrugs/special_issues/_NPFDS).

For citation purposes, cite each article independently as indicated on the article page online and as indicated below:

LastName, A.A.; LastName, B.B.; LastName, C.C. Article Title. *Journal Name* **Year**, *Volume Number*, Page Range.

ISBN 978-3-0365-3683-5 (Hbk)
ISBN 978-3-0365-3684-2 (PDF)

Cover image courtesy of Liyan Wang

© 2022 by the authors. Articles in this book are Open Access and distributed under the Creative Commons Attribution (CC BY) license, which allows users to download, copy and build upon published articles, as long as the author and publisher are properly credited, which ensures maximum dissemination and a wider impact of our publications.

The book as a whole is distributed by MDPI under the terms and conditions of the Creative Commons license CC BY-NC-ND.

Contents

About the Editor vii

Preface to "Natural Product from the Deep Sea" ix

Mingqiong Li, Saini Li, Jinhua Hu, Xiaoxia Gao, Yanlin Wang, Zhaoming Liu and Weimin Zhang
Thioester-Containing Benzoate Derivatives with α-Glucosidase Inhibitory Activity from the Deep-Sea-Derived Fungus *Talaromyces indigoticus* FS688
Reprinted from: *Mar. Drugs* **2022**, *20*, 33, doi:10.3390/md20010033 1

Hongxu Li, Xinyi Liu, Xiaofan Li, Zhangli Hu and Liyan Wang
Novel Harziane Diterpenes from Deep-Sea Sediment Fungus *Trichoderma* sp. SCSIOW21 and Their Potential Anti-Inflammatory Effects
Reprinted from: *Mar. Drugs* **2021**, *19*, 689, doi:10.3390/md19120689 11

Lu-Lu Guo, Shao-Lu Wang, Fang-Chao Zhu, Feng Xue and Li-Sheng He
Characteristics of Two Crustins from *Alvinocaris longirostris* in Hydrothermal Vents
Reprinted from: *Mar. Drugs* **2021**, *19*, 600, doi:10.3390/md19110600 23

Pei Wang, Dongyang Wang, Rongxin Zhang, Yi Wang, Fandong Kong, Peng Fu and Weiming Zhu
Novel Macrolactams from a Deep-Sea-Derived *Streptomyces* Species
Reprinted from: *Mar. Drugs* **2021**, *19*, 13, doi:10.3390/md19010013 37

Xiaojie Lu, Junjie He, Yanhua Wu, Na Du, Xiaofan Li, Jianhua Ju, Zhangli Hu, Kazuo Umezawa and Liyan Wang
Isolation and Characterization of New Anti-Inflammatory and Antioxidant Components from Deep Marine-Derived Fungus *Myrothecium* sp. Bzo-l062
Reprinted from: *Mar. Drugs* **2020**, *18*, 597, doi:10.3390/md18120597 49

Wael M. Abdel-Mageed, Lamya H. Al-Wahaibi, Burhan Lehri, Muneera S. M. Al-Saleem, Michael Goodfellow, Ali B. Kusuma, Imen Nouioui, Hariadi Soleh, Wasu Pathom-Aree, Marcel Jaspars and Andrey V. Karlyshev
Biotechnological and Ecological Potential of *Micromonospora provocatoris* sp. nov., a Gifted Strain Isolated from the Challenger Deep of the Mariana Trench
Reprinted from: *Mar. Drugs* **2021**, *19*, 243, doi:10.3390/md19050243 59

Shamsunnahar Khushi, Angela A. Salim, Ahmed H. Elbanna, Laizuman Nahar and Robert J. Capon
New from Old: Thorectandrin Alkaloids in a Southern Australian Marine Sponge, *Thorectandra choanoides* (CMB-01889)
Reprinted from: *Mar. Drugs* **2021**, *19*, 97, doi:10.3390/md19020097 79

Liyan Wang and Kazuo Umezawa
Cellular Signal Transductions and Their Inhibitors Derived from Deep-Sea Organisms
Reprinted from: *Mar. Drugs* **2021**, *19*, 205, doi:10.3390/md19040205 89

About the Editor

Kazuo Umezawa graduated from the Department of Chemistry, Faculty of Science, University of Tokyo, Japan (B.Sc.), in 1969, and from the Graduate School of Massachusetts Institute of Technology, USA (Ph.D.), in 1973. He learned medicine in Lincoln College, Oxford University, United Kingdom, and graduated with a B.A. in 1976 and an M.A. in 1979. After working at the University of Tokyo and the Institute of Microbial Chemistry, Tokyo, he became a Professor at the Department of Applied Chemistry, Faculty of Science and Technology, Keio University, in 1989, where he worked until 2012. Since 2012, he has been a Professor at the Department of Molecular Target Medicine, Aichi Medical University School of Medicine, Aichi, Japan. He is now also a Visiting Professor in Jozef Stefan International Postgraduate School, Ljubljana, Slovenia, Faculty of Health Sciences, Hokkaido University School of Medicine, Japan, and Bashkortostan State Medical University, Ufa, Russia. He received the Fukuzawa Prize from Keio University in 2011. His research interests include: the screening of cell signaling inhibitors from nature and by molecular design; the development of chemotherapeutic agents, and the mechanistic study of diseases with cell signaling inhibitors. He discovered a potent and specific inhibitor of NF-kappa B called DHMEQ in 2000. A DHMEQ ointment is now being developed in China for the treatment of severe skin inflammations and DHMEQ intraperitoneal therapy in Russia for the treatment of cancer.

Preface to "Natural Product from the Deep Sea"

Many scientists have tried to isolate novel and active compounds mainly from micro-organisms, including bacteria, Streptomyces, fungi, plants, and ordinary marine organisms since the middle of the 20th century. However, after the long history of screening, it is becoming difficult to find novel compounds anywhere in the world.

Until now, more than 28,600 marine natural products have been reported. However, with the development of marine natural products research, the hit rate of new compounds is also decreasing. Scientists are turning their attention to the deep sea. By 2008, almost 400 compounds were isolated from deep-sea organisms. By 2013, a further 188 new deep-sea natural products were reported. About 75% of the deep-sea-origin compounds were reported to show biological activity (i.e., 141 of 188 compounds), with almost half (i.e., 81 of 188 compounds) exhibiting potent cytotoxicity in human cancer cell lines [1].

In addition to the micro-organisms, there are also sponges and corals in the deep sea. An investigation of the extracts of 65 twilight-zone (50–1000 m depth) sponges, gorgonians, hard corals, and sponge-associated bacteria resulted in an extremely high hit rate (42%) of active extracts, with a hit rate for sponge and gorgonian extracts of 72% [2,3].

Therefore, deep-sea organisms are important sources of natural products, especially for screening pharmacologically active compounds. In this Special Issue, I tried to bring together articles on the screening of new bioactive metabolites produced by deep-sea organisms.

This issue includes seven original articles and one review article. Li, Zhang et al. isolated unusual thioester-containing benzoate derivatives from deep-sea derived fungus. One of them showed α-glucosidase inhibitory activity (Chapter 1). Li, Wang et al. isolated new and reported harziane-type diterpene derivatives from the deep-sea sediment-derived fungus. One of them inhibited LPS-induced NO formation in macrophage-like cells (Chapter 2). Crustins are characterized by the existence of an acidic protein domain, and they often show anti-bacterial activity. Guo et al. found two new crustins from hydrothermal vent shrimps, and one of them inhibited antibiotic-resistant Gram-negative bacteria (Chapter 3). Wang and Zhu isolated new polyene macrolactams from deep-sea sediment-derived Streptomyces. They showed antifungal activity against Candida albicans (Chapter 4). Lu et al. isolated new 2-benzoyl tetrahydrofuran enantiomers, 1S-myrothecol and 1R-myrothecol, from cultures of the deep-sea fungus. These new compounds showed cellular anti-inflammatory and anti-oxidant activities (Chapter 5). Abdel-Mageed et al. isolated n-acetylglutaminyl glutamine amide and desferrioxamine B from a Micromonospora strain collected from deep-sea of Mariana Trench (Chapter 6). Khushi et al. isolated a new tryptophan-derived alkaloid thorectandrin A from a sponge Thorectandra choanoides collected at a depth of 45 m (Chapter 7). Finally, disease-related cellular signal transductions and their inhibitors from the deep sea were reviewed (Chapter 8).

Screening of bioactive metabolites from deep-sea organisms is promising but still not popular. I would like to thank all the authors for their contribution. This Special Issue, "Natural Products from the Deep Sea", should be useful for the screening of novel and useful compounds from nature.

References

1. Skropeta, D.; Wei, L. Recent advances in deep-sea natural products. *Nat. Prod. Rep.* **2014**, *31*, 999–1025.
2. Schupp, P.J.; Kohlert-Schupp, C.; Whitefield, S.; Engemann, A.; Rohde, S.; Hemscheidt, T.; Pezzuto, J.M.; Kondratyuk, T.P.; Park, E.-J.; Marler, L.; Rostama, B.; Wright, A.D. Cancer chemopreventive and anticancer evaluation of extracts and fractions from marine macro- and microorganisms collected from Twilight Zone waters around Guam. *Nat. Prod. Commun.* **2009**, *4*, 1717–1728.
3. Wright, A.D.; Schupp. P.J.; Schrör, J.P.; Engemann, A.; Rohde, S.; Kelman, D.; de Voogd, N.; Carroll, A.; Motti, C.A. Twilight zone sponges from Guam yield theonellin isocyanate and psammaplysins I and J. *J. Nat. Prod.* **2012**, *75*, 502–506.

Kazuo Umezawa
Editor

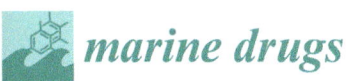

Article

Thioester-Containing Benzoate Derivatives with α-Glucosidase Inhibitory Activity from the Deep-Sea-Derived Fungus *Talaromyces indigoticus* FS688

Mingqiong Li [1,2], Saini Li [1], Jinhua Hu [1], Xiaoxia Gao [2], Yanlin Wang [3], Zhaoming Liu [1,*] and Weimin Zhang [1,*]

[1] State Key Laboratory of Applied Microbiology Southern China, Guangdong Provincial Key Laboratory of Microbial Culture Collection and Application, Institute of Microbiology, Guangdong Academy of Sciences, 100 Central Xianlie Road, Yuexiu District, Guangzhou 510070, China; LM_qiong@163.com (M.L.); lisn@gdim.cn (S.L.); m15622119835@163.com (J.H.)
[2] College of Pharmacy, Guangdong Pharmaceutical University, Guangzhou 510006, China; gaoxxia91@163.com
[3] Key Laboratory of Ocean and Marginal Sea Geology, South China Sea Institute of Oceanology, Innovation Academy of South China Sea Ecology and Environmental Engineering, Chinese Academy of Sciences, Guangzhou 510301, China; yanlinw@scsio.ac.cn
* Correspondence: liuzm@gdim.cn (Z.L.); wmzhang@gdim.cn (W.Z.)

Abstract: Eurothiocins C–H (**1–6**), six unusual thioester-containing benzoate derivatives, were isolated from the deep-sea-derived fungus *Talaromyces indigoticus* FS688 together with a known analogue eurothiocin A (**7**). Their structures were elucidated through spectroscopic analysis and the absolute configurations were determined by X-ray diffraction and ECD calculations. In addition, compound **1** exhibited significant inhibitory activity against α-glucosidase with an IC_{50} value of 5.4 µM, while compounds **4** and **5** showed moderate effects with IC_{50} values of 33.6 and 72.1 µM, respectively. A preliminary structure–activity relationship is discussed and a docking analysis was performed.

Keywords: thioester-containing benzoate; deep-sea-derived fungus; α-glucosidase inhibitory activity; docking study

1. Introduction

Organosulfur compounds, referring to sulfur-containing low-molecular-weight compounds including thiols, thioesters, and sulfoxides, continue to be a research hotspot in the field of organic chemistry due to their unique chemical properties and reactive functions [1–4]. On the one hand, sulfur is an essential element in primary metabolism from bacteria and fungi to plants and animals; for example, the cysteine is the most important amino acid in protein structures and in protein-folding pathways [5]. On the other hand, sulfur-containing secondary metabolites produced by plant, animals or microorganisms always exhibit significant biological activities such as anti-inflammatory [6], anticancer [7] and plant defense [8]. Several clinical drugs developed from natural products (NPs) are organosulfur compounds such as penicillin, cephalosporine and trabectedin (ET-743). However, sulfur-containing NPs are still relatively rare when compared to other types of NPs, and the biological significance and biosynthetic mechanisms of sulfur-containing NPs have been investigated with limited progress [7].

Since sulfur is the second most common non-metallic element, after chlorine in sea water, sulfur-containing metabolites are widely produced by different marine organisms [9]. Marine microorganisms are potential and reproducible sources of new bioactive sulfur-containing NPs, and have attracted research interest worldwide in recent years. Since the first sulfur-containing metabolite, gliovictin, was discovered from marine deuteromycete *Asteromyces cruciatus* [10], 484 non-sulfated organosulfur NPs have been isolated from marine microorganisms as of the end of 2020 and fungi contributed the most significant number of the new compounds (43%), which were reviewed by Shao C.-L. et al. [11].

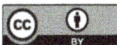

Thus, it could be concluded that marine fungi have become the most productive marine microorganisms of sulfur-containing NPs.

Deep-sea-derived fungi are a special group of microorganisms collected from sediment or water at a depth of over 1000 m. Due to their potential ability to produce novel and bioactive natural products promoted by the extreme environment, deep-sea-derived fungi have attracted considerable attention from both natural product and medicinal chemists [12]. In the course of searching for bioactive metabolites from deep-sea-derived fungi, *Talaromyces indigoticus* FS688—isolated from the South China Sea—was investigated and seven unusual thioester-containing benzoate derivatives were isolated (Figure 1). Herein, the details of the isolation, the structure identification and the biological evaluation of compounds 1–7 are discussed.

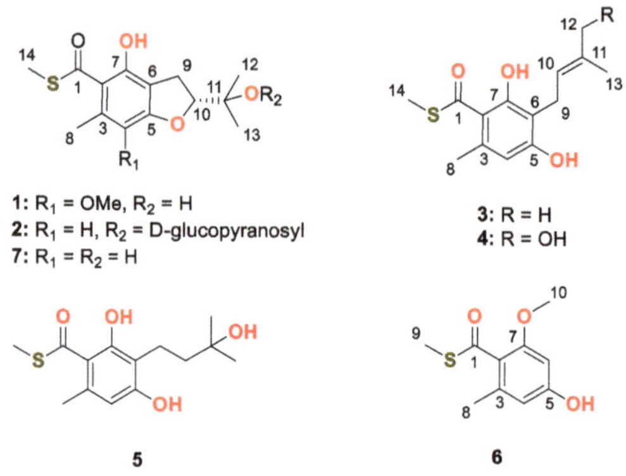

Figure 1. Chemical structures of compound 1–7.

2. Results

2.1. Structure Identification

The fermented substrate of the fungus *Talaromyces indigoticus* FS688 was extracted with ethyl acetate three times and then concentrated under reduced pressure to give a brown oil, which was further subjected to repeated silica gel with gradient elution followed by Sephdex-20 and semi-preparative HPLC purification to afford compounds 1–7 (Figure 1).

Eurothiocin C (1) was obtained as a colorless oil. The molecular formula was deduced to be $C_{15}H_{19}O_5S$ on the basis of the deprotonated quasi molecular ion peak at m/z 311.0964 $[M - H]^-$ and the characteristic ^{34}S-containing isotope ion peak at m/z 313.0938 $[M - H + 2]^-$ in a 20:1 ratio with the ^{32}S-containing ion peak from the HRESIMS spectrum. The ^1H NMR spectrum (Table 1) showed the signals of a chelating proton at δ_H 11.14 (7-OH), five singlet methyls including a methoxy group at δ_H 3.78 (Me-18), and intercoupled methylene and methine groups at δ_H 3.17/3.09 (H$_2$-9) and δ_H 4.78 (H-10), respectively. The ^{13}C NMR data resolved 15 resonances composed of six aromatic carbons, eight aliphatic carbons and a carbonyl carbon (δ_C 197.8), suggesting that a fully substituted benzene ring should be contained in compound 1. By comparing the 1D NMR data to that of the known compound eurothiocin A (7), [13] indicated that compound 1 was a methoxy additive product of eurothiocin A.

The complete structure was elucidated by analysis of 2D NMR data (Figure 2). The COSY correlations of H$_2$-9/H-10 and the HMBC correlations from H$_3$-12/H$_3$-13 to C-10/C-11 indicated the presence of an oxygenated isopentenyl unit (C-9 to C-13), which was further connected to C-6 of the benzene ring based on the correlations from H$_2$-9 to C-5, C-6 and C-7. A benzofuran core was constructed by the key HMBC correlations from H-10 to C-5. The chelating proton at 7-OH displayed HMBC correlations to C-2, C-6 and C-7, which suggested that the carbonyl group should be linked to C-2 of the benzene ring to form an intramolecular hydrogen bond. Finally, the methyl thioester moiety was deduced by the correlations from H$_3$-14 to C-1 and the characteristic chemical shifts of C-1 (δ_C 197.8), while the locations of Me-8 and 4-OMe were evaluated by the cross-peaks from H$_3$-8 to C-2/C-3/C-4 and from 4-OMe to C-4. Hence, the planar structure of compound **1** was elucidated to be a sulfur-containing benzofuran derivative as shown.

Table 1. The ^{1}H (600 MHz) and ^{13}C NMR (150 MHz) data of compounds **1**, **3** and **4**.

Position	1 [a]		3 [a]		4 [b]	
	δ_C, Type	δ_H	δ_C, Type	δ_H	δ_C, Type	δ_H
1	197.8, C		198.2, C		197.6, C	
2	116.3, C		115.4, C		115.6, C	
3	132.2, C		138.7, C		137.1, C	
4	135.8, C		111.7, CH	6.22, s	110.3, CH	6.23, s
5	156.9, C		158.9, C		158.9, C	
6	112.8, C		112.0, C		112.7, C	
7	153.2, C		160.5, C		159.0, C	
8	15.3, CH$_3$	2.59, s	25.0, CH$_3$	2.63, s	22.4, CH$_3$	2.51, s
9	28.0, CH$_2$	3.17, dd (15.6, 9.7)	22.1, CH$_2$	3.40, d (7.1)	21.0, CH$_2$	3.34, d (7.1)
		3.09, dd (15.6, 8.3)				
10	91.9, CH	4.78, dd (9.7, 8.3)	121.5, CH	5.25, tq (7.1, 1.4)	123.8, CH	5.48, brt (7.1)
11	72.0, C		135.0, C		134.0, C	
12	24.0, CH$_3$	1.24, s	25.8, CH$_3$	1.74, d (1.4)	67.7, CH$_2$	3.89, d (1.4)
13	25.7, CH$_3$	1.35, s	17.9, CH$_3$	1.81, s	12.4, CH$_3$	1.80, s
14	13.1, CH$_3$	2.46, s	13.1, CH$_3$	2.45, s	11.5, CH$_3$	2.44, s
4-OMe	60.4, CH$_3$	3.78, s				
7-OH		11.1, s		12.16, s		

[a] recorded in chloroform-d; [b] recorded in methanol-d_4.

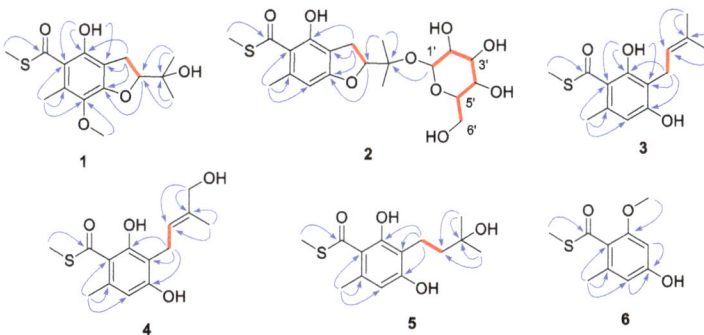

Figure 2. COSY (red bold lines) and key HMBC correlations (blue arrows) of compounds **1–6**.

Because only one chiral center was detected in **1**, the absolute configuration could be directly determined by comparing the theoretical ECD spectrum with the experimental plot. The calculated ECD spectrum of 10*R*-**1** at the PBE1PBE/tzvp level exhibited an excellent fit to the experimental plot (Figure 3), assigning the 10*R* configuration.

Eurothiocin D (**2**), obtained as a colorless oil, showed a similar 1D NMR spectrum (Table 2) to that of eurothiocin A. The main differences observed were a series of additional proton signals from δ_H 3.30 to 5.20 including an anomeric oxymethine at δ_H 5.20 and six additional carbon resonances from δ_C 61 to 94, suggesting that a glucoside moiety should be constructed in compound **2**. The COSY correlations of H-1'/H-2'/H-3'/H-4'/H-5'/H$_2$-6' confirmed the existence of the glucoside; meanwhile, the HMBC correlations (Figure 2) from H-1 to C-11 further revealed the location of the glucoside at C-11.

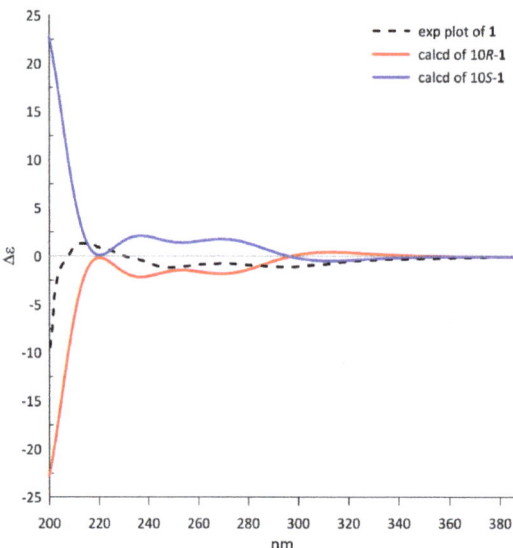

Figure 3. The calculated ECD spectra of 10*R*/10*S*-**1** at the PBE1PBE/tzvp level and the experimental plot of compound **1**.

Table 2. The ^{1}H (600 MHz) and ^{13}C NMR (150 MHz) data of compound **2**.

Position	**2** [a]				
	δ_C, Type	δ_H (J in Hz)		δ_C, Type	δ_H (J in Hz)
1	197.2, C		11	77.9, C	
2	119.8, C		12	20.5, CH$_3$	1.30, s
3	137.8, C		13	21.3, CH$_3$	1.33, s
4	103.3, CH	6.19, s	14	11.3, CH$_3$	2.43, s
5	162.9, C		1′	93.2, CH	5.20, d (3.8)
6	110.7, C		2′	72.1, CH	3.35, dd (9.8, 3.8)
7	152.6, C		3′	73.6, CH	3.54, t (9.8)
8	20.0, CH$_3$	2.32, s	4′	70.4, CH	3.30, m
9	27.7, CH$_3$	3.11, brd (3.8)	5′	72.1, CH	3.73, m
		3.13, brd (2.4)	6′	61.2, CH$_2$	3.69, m
10	89.2, CH	4.80, t (8.8)			

[a] Recorded in methanol-d_4.

The deshielded anomeric proton observed at δ_H 5.20 combined with the small $^3J_{1',2'}$ (3.8 Hz) indicated an α-glucopyranosyl linkage. Finally, the crystal of compound **2** was obtained and the X-ray diffraction analysis confirmed a α-d-glucopyranosyl unit at C-11 (Figure 4).

Eurothiocin E (**3**) was isolated as a colorless oil and gave the molecular formula $C_{14}H_{17}O_3S$ deduced by the quasi molecular ion peak at *m/z* 265.0900 [M − H]$^-$ as well as the ^{34}S-containing characteristic isotope ion peak at *m/z* 267.0879 [M − H + 2]$^-$ in a 20:1 ratio with the ^{32}S-containing ion peak from the HRESIMS spectrum. The ^{1}H NMR spectrum (Table 1) displayed the signals of a chelating proton at δ_H 12.16 (7-OH), an aromatic proton at δ_H 6.22 (H-4), an intercoupled system composed of an olefin proton (δ_H 6.22), a methylene (δ_H 3.40) and four methyls at δ_H 2.63 (Me-8), 2.45 (Me-14), 1.81 (Me-13), and 1.74 (Me-12). The ^{13}C NMR spectrum exhibited 14 signals containing eight olefinic carbons, a carboxyl carbon and five *sp*^{3} hybridized carbons. Comprehensive analysis of the 1D NMR data suggested the existence of a penta-substituted benzene ring and an exocyclic *tri*-substituted double bond in compound **3**.

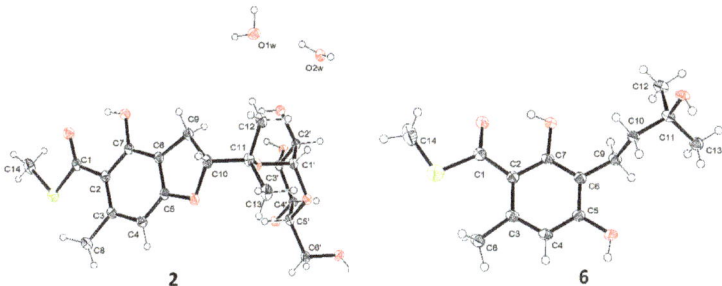

Figure 4. X-ray diffractions of compounds **2** and **6**.

The COSY correlation (Figure 2) of H$_2$-9/H-10 combined with the HMBC cross-peaks from H$_3$-12/H$_3$-13 to C-10/C-11 constructed an isopentenyl unit (C-9 to C-13), which was connected to C-6 of the benzene ring based on the correlations from H$_2$-9 to C-5/C-6/C-7. The locations of the carbonyl at C-1 and the chelating hydroxyl groups were evaluated by the HMBC correlations from 7-OH to C-2, C-6 and C-7. A similar methyl thioester moiety to that of eurothiocin C/D was deduced by the correlations from H$_3$-14 to C-1 and the characteristic chemical shifts of C-1 (δ_C 198.2). All of the above evidence indicated that compound **3** was a ring-opening precursor of eurothiocin A. Finally, the HMBC correlation (Figure 2) from H$_3$-8 to C-2/C-3/C-4 and the deshielded chemical shift of C-5 (δ_C 158.9) revealed a methyl and a hydroxy group at C-8 and C-5, respectively. Thus, the gross structure of compound **3** was established to be an isopentenyl-substituted benzoate thioester derivative.

Both eurothiocins F (**4**) and G (**5**) exhibited similar 1D NMR spectra (Tables 2 and 3) to that of compound **3**, which suggested that they are analogues containing a similar isopentenyl-substituted benzoate thioester core. Their HRESIMS spectra exhibited ^{34}S:^{32}S (20:1) isotope ion peaks. On the one hand, the main differences in compound **4** were that the methyl group (δ_H 1.74) was absent and an additional hydroxymethyl group at δ_H 3.98/δ_C 67.7 was detected, which indicated that Me-12 was oxygenated. On the other hand, in the 1D NMR spectrum of compound **5**, the signals of the *tri*-substituted double bond (Δ^{10}) were absent and the olefin proton was transferred to a methylene (δ_H 3.98/δ_C 67.7), suggesting that the Δ^{10} was hydrolyzed. Further analysis of 2D NMR spectra (Figure 2) constructed the structures of both compound **4** and **5**. The geometry of the Δ^{10} in compound **4** was deduced by the NOESY correlation (Figure S38) between H-10 and H$_2$-12; meanwhile, the structure of compound **5** was confirmed by X-ray diffraction analysis (Figure 4).

Eurothiocin H (**6**) was obtained as a colorless powder, the molecular formula of which was deduced to be C$_{10}$H$_{11}$O$_3$S based on the HRESIMS data exhibiting a quasi molecular ion peak at *m/z* 211.0435 [M − H]$^-$ and the ^{34}S-containing isotope ion peak at *m/z* 213.0412 [M − H + 2]$^-$. The methyl thioester moiety was evaluated by the characteristic methyl signals at δ_H 2.46/δ_C 12.6 and the carbonyl carbon at δ_C 195.2. A set of meta-coupled aromatic protons at δ_H 6.24/δ_H 6.27 detected in the ^{1}H NMR spectrum and six aromatic carbon signals in ^{13}C NMR revealed a benzoate thioester core in **6**. The HMBC correlations from H$_3$-8 to C-2/C-3/C-4, from H$_3$-9 to C-1, from H$_3$-10 to C-7 and from H-4/H-6 to C-2/C-5 confirmed the complete structure.

To the best of our knowledge, thioester moieties are the rarest in marine microorganisms and only 12 compounds have been discovered to date, of which seven are produced by bacteria (suncheonosides A–D [14]; nitrosporeusines A–B [15]; thiocoraline [16]), two are produced by cyanobacteria (largazole [17] and thiopalmyrone [18]) and the others were isolated from marine mollusk-derived fungi (Eurothiocins A–B [13] and N-((3R,4S)-4-methyl-2-oxotetrahydrothiophen-3-yl)acetamide [19]). This is the first report of thioester-containing NPs isolated from the deep-sea-derived fungus. In general, it is recognized that glutathione is a direct donor of the sulfur atom in sulfur-containing NPs from plants or bacteria [11]. However, how the sulfur is introduced in the biosynthesis of metabolites from fungi is still unknown. A further biosynthetic investigation will be carried out in the future to understand the biosynthesis of the thioester moieties in eurothiocins.

Table 3. The ^{1}H (600 MHz) and ^{13}C NMR (150 MHz) data of compounds **5** and **6**.

Position	5 [a]		Position	6 [b]	
	δ_C, Multiplicities	δ_H (J in Hz)		δ_C, Multiplicities	δ_H (J in Hz)
1	197.7, C		1	195.2, C	-
2	116.0, C		2	122.7, C	
3	136.5, C		3	137.8, C	
4	110.2, CH	6.23, s	4	109.1, CH	6.24, d (2.1)
5	156.9, C		5	158.3, C	
6	114.1, C		6	96.8, CH	6.27, d (2.1)
7	153.2, C		7	157.5, C	
8	22.0, CH$_3$	2.48, s	8	19.1, CH$_3$	2.24, s
9	17.5, CH$_2$	2.65, m	9	12.6, CH$_3$	2.46, s
			10	55.9, CH$_3$	3.78, s
10	41.7, CH	1.63, m			
11	70.4, C				
12	27.6, CH$_3$	1.24, s			
13	27.6, CH$_3$	1.24, s			
14	11.5, CH$_3$	2.44, s			

[a] Recorded in methanol-d_4. [b] Recorded in chloroform-d.

2.2. Bioassays and Molecular Docking

The previously reported bioactivity screening results indicated that eurothiocin A is a potential α-glucosidase inhibitor [13]. Thus, the in vitro α-glucosidase inhibitory activities of eurothiocins C–H (**1–6**) were evaluated (Table 4). Compound **2** exhibited the most significant inhibitory effect with an IC$_{50}$ value of 5.4 μM, while compounds **4** and **5** showed moderate activities with IC$_{50}$ values of 33.6 and 72.1 μM, respectively. Further, compounds **1**, **3** and **6** only displayed weak inhibitory effects at a concentration of 100 μM. The strong inhibitory effect of compound **2** might be contributed to by α-d-glucopyranosyl unit substitution at C-11, which could make it easy to interact with the enzyme. By comparing the compound with the structures and bioactivities of compounds **3–5**, it could be concluded that a hydrophilic terminal of the isopentenyl group at C-6 played an important role in inhibiting α-glucosidase. In order to predict the binding mechanism, a docking analysis of the reaction between α-glucosidase and the active compounds was performed through Autodock 4.2 (Figure 5). The protein crystallized structure of α-glucosidase from *Saccharomyces cerevisiae* was downloaded from the RSCB Protein Data Bank (pdb: 3A4A). The docking results indicated that compounds **2**, **4** and **5** bound at the same bioactive site, mainly containing the active residues Asp215, Val216, Gly217 or Ser218, which was reported by Yamamoto et al. previously [20]. Moreover, the hydrogen bonds between the 2'-OH of **2**/12-OH of **4**/11-OH of compound **5** and the residues in the site further demonstrated that the glucopyranosyl at C-11 or the hydrophilic terminal of the isopentenyl group might be the key bioactive function groups.

Table 4. α-Glucosidase inhibitory activities of compounds **1–6**.

Compounds	IC$_{50}$ (μM)
1	>100
2	5.4
3	>100
4	33.6
5	72.1
6	>100
Acarbose	317.2

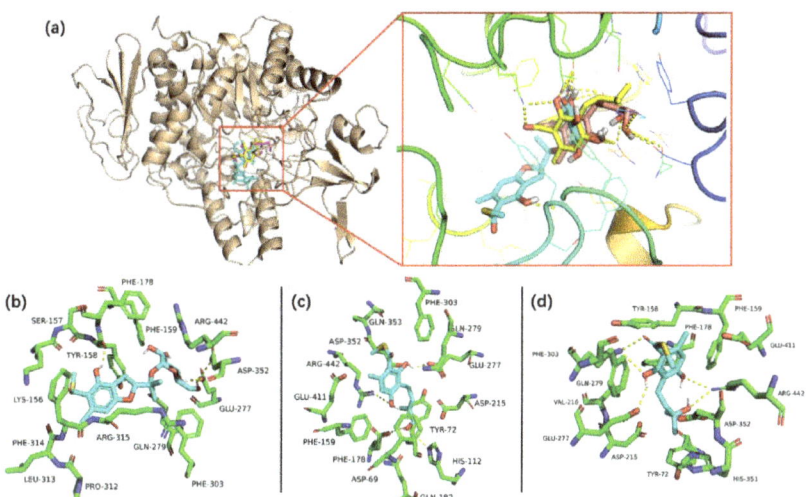

Figure 5. The complexes of compounds **1**, **4** and **5** binding in the active site of α-glucosidase (**a**) and the details of the interaction between compounds **1** (**b**), **4** (**c**), **5** (**d**) and the amino acid residue.

3. Materials and Methods

3.1. General Experimental Procedures

An Anton Paar MCP-500 (Anton Paar, Graz, Austria) and a Jasco 820 spectropolarimeter were used to measure the circular dichroism (ECD) and the UV spectra, respectively. ECD and UV spectra were recorded at the range of 200–400 nm under N_2 gas production. IR spectra were recorded on a Shimadzu IR Affinity-1 spectrophotometer. All the NMR spectra were measured on a 600 MHz Bruker Avance-III HD spectrometer and the tetramethylsilane was used as an internal standard. HR-ESI-MS was measured on a Bruker maXis high-resolution mass spectrometer. A Shimadzu LC-20 AT (equipped with an SPD-M20A PDA detector) was used for the preparative separations. The ACE 5 PFP-C_{18} column (250 × 10.0 mm, 5 µm, 12 nm) was used for semi-preparative HPLC separation and the CHIRAL-MD (2)-RH column (250 × 10.0 mm, 5 µm) was used for chiral separation (Guangzhou FLM Scientific Instrument Co., Ltd, Guangzhou, China). The commercial silica gel (SiO_2; 200–300 mesh; Qingdao Marine Chemical Plant, Qingdao, China) and Sephadex LH-20 gel (GE Healthcare Bio-Sciences ABSE-751, Uppsala, Sweden) were used for column chromatography. All solvents were of analytical grade (Guangzhou Chemical Regents Company, Ltd., Guangzhou, China). The natural sea salt was purchased from Guangdong Yueyan saltern. The α-glucosidase from *Saccharomyces cerevisiae* and *p*-nitrophenyl-α-d-glucopyranoside (*p*-NPG) used in bioassays were purchased from Sigma-Aldrich (St. Louis, MO, USA).

3.2. Fungal Material

The fungal strain FS688 was identified to be *Talaromyces indigoticus*, which was collected from deep-sea sediment in the South China Sea (118° 19.692′ N, 20° 38.982′ E; depth 2372 m) in September 2020. Fungal identification was carried out by morphological traits and ITS rDNA sequence analysis. The sequence data have been submitted to GenBank, under accession number OL774516. The strain was deposited at the Guangdong Provincial Key Laboratory of Microbial Culture Collection and Application, Institute of Microbiology, Guangdong Academy of Sciences. Working stocks were prepared on PDA (agar 4 g/L, potato 200 g/L, glucose 20 g/L, KH_2PO_4 3 g/L, $MgSO_4 \bullet 7H_2O$ 1.5 g/L, vitamin B_1 10 mg/L, natural sea salt 15 g/L) slants stored at 4 °C.

3.3. Fermentation, Extraction, and Isolation

The grown mycelia were inoculated in 250 mL of PDB culture for 5 days in a 200 rpm rotary shaker at 28 °C. Then, the culture was transferred into the rice medium (12 Erlenmeyer flasks each containing 250 g rice and 400 mL H_2O with 0.3% natural sea salt) and incubated at room temperature for another 30 days. After fermentation, the solid fermented substrate was extracted with methanol three times to obtain a dark brown oily residue (20.3 g), which was further subjected to silica gel column chromatography, eluting with petroleum ether/EtOAc in a linear gradient (9:1 to 1:9) to afford six fractions (Fr.1–Fr. 6). Compounds **3** (250 mg) and **7** (600 mg) were purified from Fr.1 by Sephdex-20 (eluting with 1:1 MeOH/CH_2Cl_2) and silica gel column (eluting with 20% petroleum ether/EtOAc), respectively. Fr.2 was subjected to repeated silica gel column chromatography, eluting with MeOH/CH_2Cl_2 to obtained crude **1**, which was further purified by HPLC equipped with a PFP-C_{18} column to obtain compounds **1** (7.2 mg, 80% MeOH/H_2O, 2 mL/min, T_R = 12.5 min), **6** (8.0 mg, 80% MeOH/H_2O, 2 mL/min, T_R = 10.5 min) and **5** (20 mg, 70% MeOH/H_2O, 2 mL/min, T_R = 25.5 min). Fr.3 was subjected to repeated silica gel column chromatography, Sephdex-20 (eluting with 50% MeOH/CH_2Cl_2) followed by HPLC with an Ar-C_{18} column to obtain compound **4** (1.6 mg, 90% MeOH/H_2O, 2 mL/min, T_R = 9.5 min). Fr. 6 was subjected to HPLC equipped with a PFP-C_{18} column to afford compound **2** (15.3 mg, 55% MeOH/H_2O, 6 mL/min, T_R = 11.4 min).

Eurothiocin C (**1**): colorless oil; $[\alpha]_D^{25}$ + 3.8 (c 0. 1, MeOH); UV (MeOH) λ_{max} (log ε): 207 (4.17), 239 (3.71), and 295 (3.35) nm; IR (KBr): 2972, 2931, 2358, 1647, 1456, 1261, 1076, 1012, and 949 cm^{-1}; ^1H and ^{13}C NMR data, Table 1. HRESIMS m/z 311.0964 [M − H]$^−$ (calcd for $C_{15}H_{19}O_5S$, 311.0959).

Eurothiocin D (**2**): colorless oil; $[\alpha]_D^{25}$ + 2.0 (c 0.1, MeOH); UV (MeOH) λ_{max} (log ε): 208 (4.17) 239 (3.72), and 295 (3.35) nm; IR (KBr): 3392, 2927, 2359, 1653, 1417, 1232, 1022, and 823 cm^{-1}; ^1H and ^{13}C NMR data, Table 2. HRESIMS m/z 443.1391 [M − H]$^−$ (calcd for $C_{20}H_{27}O_9S$, 443.1381).

Eurothiocin E (**3**): colorless oil; UV (MeOH) λ_{max} (log ε): 199 (4.15), 222 (3.68), and 283 (4.14) nm; IR (KBr): 3402, 2974, 2927, 2358, 1581, 1451, 1220, 1157, and 871 cm^{-1}; ^1H and ^{13}C NMR data, Table 1; HRESIMS m/z 265.0900 [M − H]$^−$ (calcd for $C_{14}H_{17}O_3S$, 265.0904).

Eurothiocin F (**4**): colorless powder; UV (MeOH) 201 (4.15) and 296 (3.33) nm; IR (KBr): 3408, 2924, 2361, 1635, 1456, 1417, 1232, 1024, 1002, 981, and 820 cm^{-1}; ^1H and ^{13}C NMR data, Table 1; HRESIMS m/z 281.0857, [M − H]$^−$ (calcd for $C_{14}H_{17}O_4S$, 281.0853).

Eurothiocin G (**5**): colorless oil; UV (MeOH) λ_{max} (log ε): 201 (4.18) and 296 (3.33) nm; IR (KBr): 2979, 2926, 2358, 1522, 1418, 1227, 1101, and 974 cm^{-1}; ^1H and ^{13}C NMR data, Table 3; HRESIMS m/z 307.0974 [M + Na]$^+$ (calcd for $C_{28}H_{34}NO_3$, 307.0975).

Eurothiocin H (**6**): colorless powder; UV (MeOH) λ_{max} (log ε): 204 (4.18), 227 (3.55), and 276 (4.02) nm; IR (KBr): 3392, 2927, 2854, 2359, 2341, 1602, 1456, 1338, 1155, 1091, 1022, and 899 cm^{-1}; ^1H and ^{13}C NMR data, Table 3. HRESIMS m/z 211.0435 [M − H]$^−$ (calcd for $C_{10}H_{11}O_3S$, 211.0434).

Crystal diffraction data of compound **2**: Data were collected on an Agilent Xcalibur Nova single-crystal diffractometer using Cu Kα radiation. The crystal structure was refined by full-matrix least-squares calculation with the SHELXT. Crystallographic data have been deposited in the Cambridge Crystallographic Data Centre (deposition number: CCDC 2126903). Crystal data: $C_{20}H_{32}O_{11}S$ (M = 480.51); block crystal (0.1 × 0.08 × 0.06); space group P212121; unit cell dimensions a = 7.0695(1) Å, b = 7.9635(1) Å, c = 40.8016(6) Å, α = 90°, β = 90°, γ = 90°, V = 2297.05(6) Å^3, and Z = 4; T = 100.0(1) K; ρ_{cald} = 1.389 mg/m^3; absorption coefficient 1.765 mm^{-1}; F(000) = 1024, a total of 11418 reflections were collected in the range 4.334° < θ < 74.356°, independent reflections 4535 [R(int) = 0.0269]; the number of data/parameters/restraints were 4535/0/318; goodness of fit on F^2 = 0.957; final R indices [I > 2σ(I)] R_1 = 0.0348 and wR_2 = 0.1111; R indices (all data) R_1 = 0.0368 and wR_2 = 0.1129.

Crystal diffraction data of compound **5**: The conditions of data collection and program of refinement were the same as that of compound **2**. Crystallographic data have been deposited in the Cambridge Crystallographic Data Centre (deposition number: CCDC 2126902). Crystal data: $C_{14}H_{20}O_4S$ (M = 284.36); block crystal (0.20 × 0.15 × 0.10); space group P21/c; unit cell dimensions a = 6.1047(3) Å, b = 29.7526(14) Å, c = 8.0597(4) Å, α = 90°, β = 108.996(6)°, γ = 90°, V = 1384.17(13) Å^3, and Z = 4; T = 100.0(1) K; ρ_{cald} = 1.365 mg/m^3; absorption coefficient 2.155 mm^{-1}; F(000) = 608, a total of 6484 reflections were collected in the range 5.449° < θ < 74.170°, independent reflections 2664 [R(int) = 0.0490]; the number of data/parameters/restraints were 2664/0/179; goodness of fit on F^2 = 1.090; final R indices [I > 2σ(I)] R_1 = 0.0819 and ωR_2 = 0.2060; R indices (all data) R_1 = 0.1036 and ωR_2 = 0.2162.

3.4. Details of Quantum Chemical Calculations

Spartan'14 software (Wavefunction Inc.) and the Gaussian 09 program were used for the Merck molecular force field (MMFF) and DFT/TD-DFT calculations, respectively [21]. Conformers with an energy window lower the 10 kcal mol^{-1} from MMFF calculations were generated and re-optimized at the b3lyp/6-31+g(d,p) level, and the frequency calculations were carried out at the same level to estimate their relative thermal free energy (ΔG) at 298.15 K. Finally, conformers with the Boltzmann distribution over 5% were chosen for energy calculations at the b3lyp/6-311+g(d,p) level (rotatory strengths for a total of 20 excited states were calculated). The solvent effects were considered based on the self-consistent reaction field (SCRF) method with the polarizable continuum model (PCM). The final spectra were generated by the SpecDis program [22] using a Gaussian band shape with a 0.30 eV exponential half-width from dipole-length dipolar and rotational strengths.

3.5. α-Glucosidase Inhibition Assay

The method used for the α-glucosidase inhibitory activity assay was based on previously reported literature with slight modification [23]. The pre-reaction mixture consisted of 130 μL of PBS (100 mM, pH 7.0), 30 μL of enzyme (1 U/mL) and 0.5 μL of the test compounds at different concentrations. After incubation at 37 °C for 10 min, 40 μL of *p*NPG was added and the mixture was further incubated at 37 °C for 15 min. Finally, the absorbance was measured at 405 nm on an automatic microplate reader. Acarbose was used as the positive control (IC_{50} = 317.2 μM). All experiments were carried out in triplicate.

3.6. Docking Analysis

The minimized structure of compound **2** was obtained from X-ray diffraction, while the preferred structures of compounds **4** and **5** were optimized by Spartan'14 software based on the MMFF. The energy grid maps for each atom type in the ligands as well as the electrostatic and de-solvation maps were calculated using the AutoGrid 4.2.6 program. The docking analysis was carried out in Autodock Tools package v1.5.4 (ADT, http://mgltools.scripps.edu/, 17 December 2021) based on a previously reported method. The docking pose was placed in a grid box of 90 × 90 × 90 Å^3 (0.375 Å of grid spacing) with the protein at the center of the box [23]. The results were analyzed by ADT and the figures were prepared with PyMOL visualization tool (v1.7.4, Schrödinger, New York, NY, USA).

Supplementary Materials: The following supporting information can be downloaded at: https://www.mdpi.com/article/10.3390/md20010033/s1, Figures S1–S31. The NMR spectra of compounds **1–6**; Figures S32–S37. The HRESIMS spectra of compounds **1–6**; Figure S38. The key NOE correlation of compound **4**; Table S1. Energy analysis for the conformers of 10R-**1**.

Author Contributions: Chemical experiments, M.L. and J.H.; biological investigation, S.L.; fungal resources, Y.W.; data curation, Z.L. and W.Z.; writing—original draft preparation, Z.L.; writing—review and editing, X.G. and W.Z.; funding acquisition, Z.L. and W.Z. All authors have read and agreed to the published version of the manuscript.

Funding: This research was funded by National Natural Science Foundation of China (41906106, 31272087, 41876052), the GDAS' Project of Science and Technology Development (2019GDASYL-0103007), Guangdong Provincial Special Fund for Marine Economic Development Project (GDNRC [2020]042) and the Guangdong MEDP fund (GDOE [2019]A35). Data and samples were collected onboard of R/V "JiaGeng" implementing the open research cruise NORC2019-06 and NORC2020-06 supported by NSFC Shiptime Sharing Project (41849906 and 41949906).

Data Availability Statement: Data are contained within the article or Supplementary Material.

Acknowledgments: We thank the Computing Center of the Chinese Academy of Sciences; Ai-Jun Sun, Yun Zhang and Xuan Ma, the South China Sea Institute of Oceanology, and the Chinese Academy of Sciences, for the measurement of HRESIMS and X-ray diffractions. We gratefully acknowledge support from the Guangzhou Branch of the Super.

Conflicts of Interest: The authors declare no conflict of interest.

References

1. Ilardi:, E.A.; Vitaku, E.; Njardarson, J.T. Data-mining for sulfur and fluorine: An evaluation of pharmaceuticals to reveal opportunities for drug design and discovery. *J. Med. Chem.* **2014**, *57*, 2832–2842. [CrossRef]
2. Feng, M.; Tang, B.; Liang, S.H.; Jiang, X. Sulfur containing scaffolds in drugs: Synthesis and application in medicinal chemistry. *Curr. Top. Med. Chem.* **2016**, *16*, 1200–1216. [CrossRef]
3. Scott, K.A.; Njardarson, J.T. Analysis of US FDA-approved drugs containing sulfur atoms. *Top. Curr. Chem.* **2018**, *376*, 5. [CrossRef] [PubMed]
4. Milito, A.; Brancaccio, M.; D'Argenio, G.; Castellano, I. Natural sulfur-containing compounds: An alternative therapeutic strategy against liver fibrosis. *Cells* **2019**, *8*, 1356. [CrossRef]
5. Brosnan, J.T.; Brosnan, M.E. The sulfur-containing amino acid: An overview. *J. Nutri.* **2006**, *136*, 1636–1640. [CrossRef]
6. Cao, X.; Cao, L.; Zhang, W.; Lu, R.; Bian, J.-S.; Nie, X. Therapeutic potential of sulfur-containing natural products in inflammatory diseases. *Pharmacol. Therapeut.* **2020**, *216*, 107678. [CrossRef]
7. Pan, C.; Kuranaga, T.; Liu, C.; Lu, S.; Shinzato, N.; Kakeya, H. Thioamycolamides A–E, sulfur-containing cycliclipopeptides produced by the rare Actinomycete *Amycolatopsis* sp. *Org. Lett.* **2020**, *8*, 3014–3017. [CrossRef]
8. Abdalla, M.A.; Mühling, K.H. Plant-derived sulfur containing natural products produced as a response to biotic and abiotic stresses: A review of their structural diversity and medicinal importance. *J. App. Bot. Food Qual.* **2019**, *92*, 204–215.
9. Jimenez, C. Marine sulfur-containing natural products. *Stud. Nat. Prod. Chem.* **2001**, *25*, 811–917.
10. Shin, J.; Fenical, W. Isolation of gliovictin from the marine deuteromycete *Asteromyces cruciatus*. *Phytochemistry* **1987**, *26*, 3347. [CrossRef]
11. Hai, Y.; Wei, M.-Y.; Wang, C.-Y.; Gu, Y.-C.; Shao, C.-L. The intriguing chemistry and biology of sulfur-containing natural products from marine microorganisms (1987–2020). *Mar. Life Sci. Technol.* **2021**, *3*, 488–518. [CrossRef]
12. Wang, Y.-T.; Xue, Y.-R.; Liu, C.-H. A brief review of bioactive metabolites derived from deep-sea fungi. *Mar. Drugs* **2015**, *13*, 4594–4616. [CrossRef]
13. Liu, Z.; Xia, G.; Chen, S.; Liu, Y.; Li, H.; She, Z. Eurothiocin A and B, sulfur-containing benzofurans from a soft coral-derived fungus *Eurotium rubrum* SH-823. *Mar. Drugs* **2014**, *12*, 3669–3680. [CrossRef] [PubMed]
14. Shin, B.; Ahn, S.; Noh, M.; Shin, J.; Oh, D.C. Suncheonosides A–D, benzothioate glycosides from a marine-derived Streptomyces sp. *J. Nat. Prod.* **2015**, *78*, 1390–1396. [CrossRef]
15. Yang, A.G.; Si, L.L.; Shi, Z.P.; Tian, L.; Liu, D.; Zhou, D.M.; Proksch, P.; Lin, W.H. Nitrosporeusines A and B, unprecedented thioester–bearing alkaloids from the Arctic *Streptomyces nitrosporeus*. *Org. Lett.* **2013**, *15*, 5366–5369. [CrossRef]
16. Perez Baz, J.; Cañedo, L.M.; Fernández Puentes, J.L.; Silva Elipe, M.V. Thiocoraline, a novel depsipeptide with antitumor activity produced by a marine Micromonospora. II. Physico-chemical properties and structure determination. *J. Antibiot.* **1997**, *50*, 738–741.
17. Taori, K.; Paul, V.J.; Luesch, H. Structure and activity of largazole, a potent antiproliferative agent from the foridian marine cyanobacterium *Symploca* sp. *J. Am. Chem. Soc.* **2008**, *130*, 1806–1807. [CrossRef]
18. Pereira, A.R.; Etzbach, L.; Engene, N.; Muller, R.; Gerwick, W.H. Molluscicidal metabolites from an assemblage of palmyra atoll cyanobacteria. *J. Nat. Prod.* **2011**, *74*, 1175–1181. [CrossRef]
19. Han, X.; Li, P.; Luo, X.; Qian, D.; Tang, X.; Li, G. Two new compounds from the marine sponge derived fungus Penicillium chrysogenum. *Nat. Prod. Res.* **2019**, *34*, 2926–2930. [CrossRef]
20. Yamamoto, K.; Nakayama, A.; Yamamoto, Y.; Tabata, S. Val216 decides the substrate specificity of α-glucosidase in Saccharomyces cerevisiae. *Eur. J. Biochem.* **2004**, *271*, 3414–3420. [CrossRef]
21. Frisch, M.J.; Trucks, G.W.; Schlegel, H.B.; Scuseria, G.E.; Robb, M.A.; Cheeseman, J.R.; Scalmani, G.; Barone, V.; Mennucci, B.; Petersson, G.A.; et al. *Gaussian 09, Revision D.01*; Gaussian, Inc.: Wallingford, CT, USA, 2013.
22. Bruhn, T.; Schaumlöffel, A.; Hemberger, Y.; Bringmann, G. SpecDis: Quantifying the comparison of calculated and experimental electronic circular dichroism spectra. *Chirality* **2013**, *25*, 243–249. [CrossRef]
23. Fan, J.; Kuang, Y.; Dong, Z.; Yi, Y.; Zhou, Y.; Li, B.; Qiao, X.; Ye, M. Prenylated Phenolic Compounds from the Aerial Parts of *Glycyrrhiza uralensis* as PTP1B and α-Glucosidase Inhibitors. *J. Nat. Prod.* **2020**, *83*, 814–824. [CrossRef]

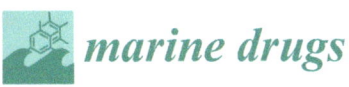

Article

Novel Harziane Diterpenes from Deep-Sea Sediment Fungus *Trichoderma* sp. SCSIOW21 and Their Potential Anti-Inflammatory Effects

Hongxu Li [1,2], Xinyi Liu [1], Xiaofan Li [1,*], Zhangli Hu [1,2] and Liyan Wang [1,*]

[1] Shenzhen Key Laboratory of Marine Bioresource and Eco-Environmental Science, College of Life Sciences and Oceanography, Shenzhen University, Shenzhen 518060, China; lhx@szu.edu.cn (H.L.); 2060251016@email.szu.edu.cn (X.L.); huzl@szu.edu.cn (Z.H.)
[2] Key Laboratory of Optoelectronic Engineering, Shenzhen University, Shenzhen 518060, China
* Correspondence: lixiaof@szu.edu.cn (X.L.); lwang@szu.edu.cn (L.W.); Tel.: +86-755-2601-2653 (L.W.)

Abstract: Five undescribed harziane-type diterpene derivatives, namely harzianol K (**1**), harzianol L (**4**), harzianol M (**5**), harzianol N (**6**), harzianol O (**7**), along with two known compounds, hazianol J (**2**) and harzianol A (**3**) were isolated from the deep-sea sediment-derived fungus *Trichoderma* sp. SCSIOW21. The relative configurations were determined by meticulous spectroscopic methods including 1D, 2D NMR spectroscopy, and HR-ESI-MS. The absolute configurations were established by the ECD curve calculations and the X-ray crystallographic analysis. These compounds (**1**, and **4–7**) contributed to increasing the diversity of the caged harziane type diterpenes with highly congested skeleton characteristics. Harzianol J (**2**) exhibited a weak anti-inflammatory effect with 81.8% NO inhibition at 100 μM.

Keywords: *Trichoderma*; harziane diterpenes; NO inhibition

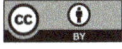

1. Introduction

The *Trichoderma* fungus, widely distributed in terrestrial and marine habitats, is a kind of important renewable natural resource with high economic value and application prospects. Among them, the species in the marine environment, together with *Penicillium* and *Aspergillus*, contributed to the discovery of more than half of the new terpenoids from marine fungi [1,2]. However, *Trichoderma* was rarely reported from deep marine ecosystems. During 2013 to 2019, a total of 151 novel compounds were reported from deep marine derived-fungi, of which 41.2% were from *Penicillium*, 28.1% were from *Aspergillus*, while only 1 *Trichoderma* was reported from the deep marine system [1].

Harziane-type diterpenes, containing unique tetracyclic 6-5-4-7 carbon skeleton with 5–6 contiguous stereocenters, are rarely encountered in other organisms. The unprecedented skeleton was initially discovered in 1992 from *Trichoderma harzianum* Rifai [3]. To date, only 44 harziane diterpenes have been reported, almost all of which were discovered solely from *Trichoderma* sp., except for heteroscyphsic acid A from Chinese liverwort *Heteroscyphus coalitus* [4]. These compounds exhibited extensive bioactivities, including anti-bacterial [5–10], cytotoxic [8,11–13], anti-inflammatory [13,14], anti-HIV [14], phytotoxic [15], algicidal [5,7,16,17], and marine zooplankton toxic activities [6,16] (Table S1 and Figure S1).

During our ongoing investigations on inhibitors from deep-sea fungi [18–23] against nitric oxide (NO) production induced by lipopolysaccharide (LPS), *Trichoderma* sp. SC-SIOW21, which was isolated from sea sediment at a depth of over 1000 m, was found to be active. The subsequent cultivation of this strain resulted in the isolation of seven harziane diterpenes, including five new compounds. Herein, we report the isolation and identification procedures, as well as the anti-inflammatory, anti-fungal, and anti-bacterial activities of these compounds.

2. Results and Discussion

The fungus *Trichoderma* sp. SCSIOW21 was cultured at room temperature under static conditions. The BuOH extraction was fractioned and purified by silica gel, medium pressure ODS column chromatography, and semi-preparative HPLC to obtain seven harziane diterpenes (Figure 1).

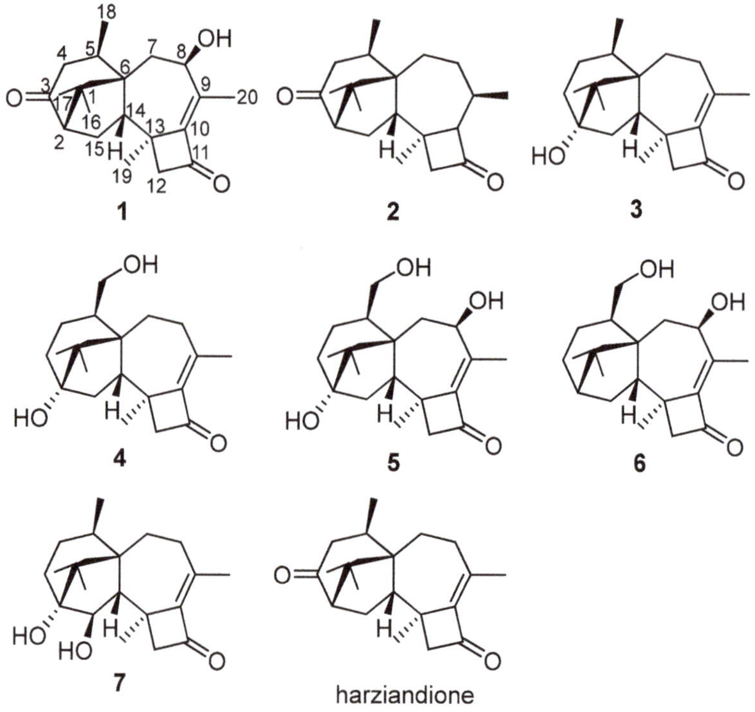

Figure 1. Compounds 1–7 and harziandione.

Compound **1** was isolated as colorless crystal, with molecular formula as $C_{20}H_{28}O_3$ using HRESIMS data. The IR spectrum showed strong absorption bands for two carbonyl groups at 1734 and 1695 cm^{-1}, which was consistent with those reported for harziandione [3]. The ^{1}H NMR and ^{13}C NMR spectroscopy spectra along with HSQC data suggested five methyls, four methylenes, four methines, and seven quaternary carbon atoms (Tables 1 and 2). The above NMR spectroscopy signal pattern was similar to the prior report for harziandione [3], except for 3 major differences: an additional hydroxy group at δ 5.31, an absent methylene group, and an extra hydroxy group at δ 4.24 compared with harziandione. The up-field shifts of H-8 to δ 4.24 and C-8 to δ 72.4 suggested this group connected to C-8 (Tables 1 and 2). ^{1}H-^{1}H COSY correlations between 8-OH and H-8, H-8 and H-7, as well as HMBC correlations from 8-OH to C-8 and C-7 also confirmed the elucidation (Figure 2). This conclusion was further secured by careful analysis of 1D, 2D NMR spectroscopy data, and compound **1** was named as harzianol K, with the molecular framework shown in Figure 2.

Table 1. ^{1}H NMR spectroscopy (600 MHz) [a] of compounds **1**, **4–7**.

No.	1 δ_H (J in Hz)	4 δ_H (J in Hz)	5 δ_H (J in Hz)	6 δ_H (J in Hz)	7 δ_H (J in Hz)
1					
2	2.06, d (8.0)			2.26, dd (11.0, 8.0)	
2-OH		4.17, s	4.14, s		
3α		1.81, m [b]	1.77, m	1.78, m	1.80, m
3β		1.32, dd (12.0, 7.0)	1.30, dd (12.0, 7.0)	1.23, m	1.31, m [b]
4α	2.92, dd (17.0, 11.0)	1.80, m	1.85, m	1.89, m	1.85, m
4β	1.84, d (17.0)	1.64, d (12.0)	1.60, m	1.48, dd (14.0, 6.0)	1.34, m
5	3.38, m	2.13, t (8.0)	2.71, t (8.0)	2.75, t (8.0)	2.32, m [b]
6					
7α	2.16, dd (15.0, 5.0)	1.76, m [b]	2.11, dd (15.0, 5.0)	2.14, dd (15.0, 5.0)	2.35, m [b]
7β	1.36, dd (15.0, 2.0)	1.28, m	1.36, dd (15.0, 2.0)	1.30, dd (15.0, 2.0)	1.90, ddd (13.0, 7.0, 2.0)
8α	4.24, d (5.0, 2.0)	2.52, m	4.21, dd (5.0, 2.0)	4.22, dd (5.0, 2.0)	1.98, dd (13.0, 7.0)
8β		1.88, ddd (16.0, 6.0, 2.0)			1.29, m [b]
8-OH	5.31, brs		5.45, brs		
9					
10					
11					
12α	2.77, d (16.0)	2.60, d (16.0)	2.65, d (16.0)	2.71, d (16.0)	2.98, d (16.0)
12β	2.33, d (16.0)	2.26, d (16.0)	2.29, d (16.0)	2.33, d (16.0)	2.34, d (16.0)
13					
14	2.57, dd (11.0, 9.0)	2.21, dd (12.0, 9.0)	2.33, dd (12.0, 9.0)	1.56, m	2.07, d (6.0)
15α	1.98, m	1.58, dd (13.0, 9.0)	1.65, m	1.84, m	3.65, d (6.0)
15β	1.49, dd (14.0, 9.0)	1.69, dd (13.0,12.0)	1.57, m	1.35, m	
16	0.93, s	0.81, s	0.82, s	0.80, s	0.84, s
17	0.91, s	0.66, s	0.70, s	0.84, s	0.89, s
18α	1.18, d (7.0)	3.41, m	3.85, d (10.0)	3.89, d (10.0)	0.99, d (7.0)
18β		3.28, m	3.23, m	3.26, m	
18-OH		4.39, t (6.0)			
19	1.53, s	1.39, s	1.46, s	1.51, s	1.43, s
20	2.04, s	2.01, s	2.03, s	2.03, s	2.02, s

[a] Recorded in DMSO-d_6; [b] overlapped signals.

Table 2. ^{13}C NMR spectroscopy (150 MHz) [a] data of Compounds **1**, **4–7**.

No.	1 δ_C, Type	4 δ_C, Type	5 δ_C, Type	6 δ_C, Type	7 δ_C, Type
1	50.5, C	48.5, C	49.2, C	51.1, C	48.2, C
2	58.9, CH	77.9, C	77.4, C	51.8, CH	75.9, C
3	213.6, C	33.2, CH$_2$	33.5, CH$_2$	25.5, CH$_2$	30.4, CH$_2$
4	43.2, CH$_2$	22.6, CH$_2$	23.9, CH$_2$	22.0, CH$_2$	25.2, CH$_2$
5	31.4, CH	40.1, CH	41.7, CH	42.4, CH	27.5, CH
6	51.7, C	52.7, C	53.1, C	45.7, C	50.7, C
7	33.0, CH$_2$	30.2, CH$_2$	34.3, CH$_2$	33.7, CH$_2$	29.3, CH$_2$
8	72.4, CH	29.3, CH$_2$	73.5, CH	73.1, CH	31.5, CH$_2$
9	144.4, C	145.5, C	143.0, C	143.1, C	145.8, C
10	150.4, C	149.7, C	150.0, C	150.6, C	149.6, C
11	199.6, C	198.2, C	200.0, C	200.1, C	198.2, C
12	58.8, CH$_2$	59.2, CH$_2$	58.9, CH$_2$	58.9, CH$_2$	59.1, CH$_2$
13	40.1, C	40.0, C	40.7, C	40.9, C	40.0, C
14	52.2, CH$_2$	50.6, CH	50.5, CH	42.4, CH	60.1, CH
15	26.1, CH	35.6, CH$_2$	35.7, CH$_2$	27.1, CH$_2$	73.5, CH
16	25.6, CH$_3$	19.7, CH$_3$	20.1, CH$_3$	25.8, CH$_3$	20.5, CH$_3$
17	23.4, CH$_3$	18.9, CH$_3$	19.0, CH$_3$	21.9, CH$_3$	19.7, CH$_3$
18	22.8, CH$_3$	63.9, CH$_2$	65.6, CH$_2$	65.9, CH$_2$	19.9, CH$_3$
19	20.2, CH$_3$	21.6, CH$_3$	21.0, CH$_3$	21.0, CH$_3$	22.3, CH$_3$
20	20.1, CH$_3$	22.0, CH$_3$	20.2, CH$_3$	20.2, CH$_3$	21.9, CH$_3$

[a] Recorded in DMSO-d_6.

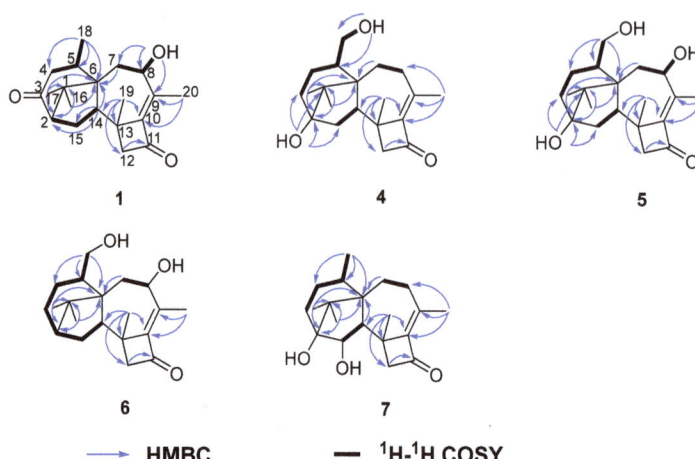

Figure 2. Key 2D NMR spectroscopy correlations of compounds **1** and **4–7**.

The relative configuration of **1** was determined by ^{1}H-^{1}H ROESY spectrum. The ^{1}H-^{1}H correlations—H-14 and H-2, H-14 and Me-16, H-5 and Me-19, Me-18 and 8-OH—indicated that H-2, H-14, Me-16, Me-17, and Me-18 were located on one side of the molecule, whereas Me-19 and H-5 were located on the opposite side (Figure 3).

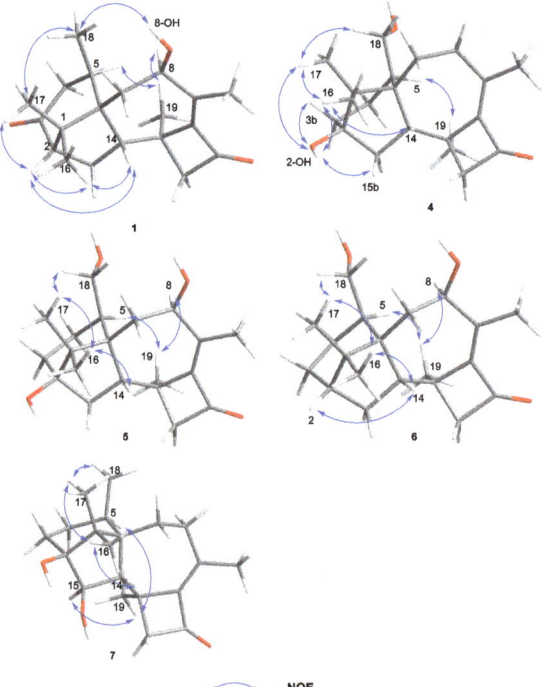

Figure 3. Key NOE correlations of compounds **1** and **4–7**.

The experimental CD spectrum of **1** was in accordance with the theoretically calculated ECD curve of the 2*S*, 5*R*, 6*R*, 8*S*, 13*S*, and 14*S* configuration. A total of 3 cotton effects were observed at 245 nm (negative), 292 nm (positive), and 351 nm (positive) (Figure 4a). Eventually, the stereocenters of **1** were determined as 2*S*, 5*R*, 6*R*, 8*S*, 13*S*, and 14*S* unambiguously through analysis of X-ray single-crystallography (Figure 5).

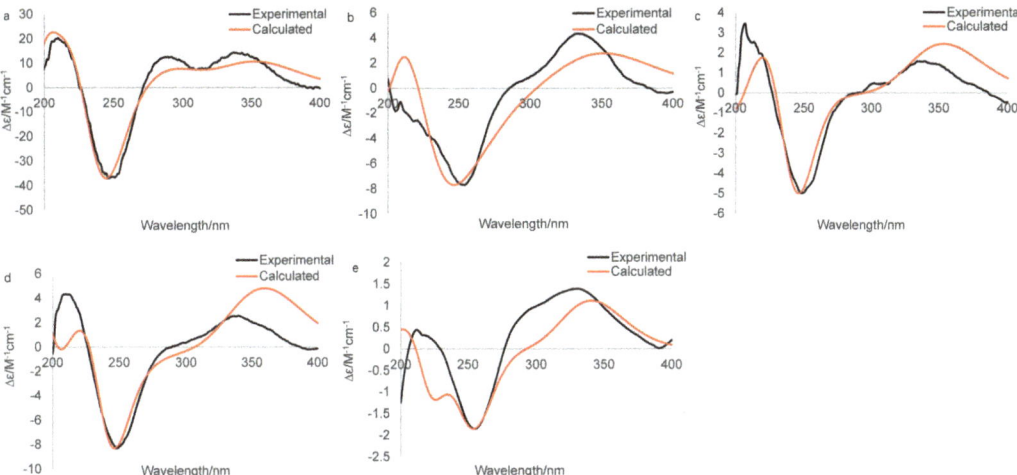

Figure 4. Experimental and calculated (for 2*S*, 5*R*, 6*R*, 8*S*, 13*S*, 14*S*) ECD spectra of **1** (**a**), experimental and calculated (for 2*S*, 5*R*, 6*R*, 13*S*, 14*S*) ECD spectra of **4** (**b**), experimental and calculated (for 2*S*, 5*R*, 6*R*, 8*S*, 13*S*, 14*S*) ECD spectra of **5** (**c**), experimental and calculated (for 2*S*, 5*R*, 6*R*, 8*S*, 13*S*, 14*S*) ECD spectra of **6** (**d**), Experimental and calculated (for 2*S*, 5*R*, 6*R*, 13*S*, 14*S*, 15*S*) ECD spectra of **7** (**e**).

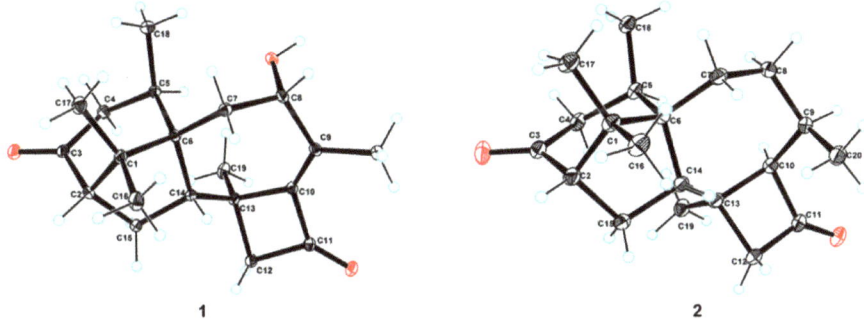

Figure 5. X-ray single-crystallography structures of **1** and **2**. The ellipsoids of non-hydrogen atoms are shown at 30% probability levels for crystal structures.

Compounds **2** and **3** were confirmed as known compounds, namely harzianol J [8] and harzianol A [13], by comparing their NMR spectroscopy data with those reported in the literature (Tables S2 and S3) [8]. Nevertheless, the absolute configuration of **2** was not determined previously. Herein we report it as 2*S*, 5*R*, 6*R*, 13*S*, and 14*S* by X-ray diffraction (Figure 5).

Compounds **4–7** were all purified as colorless gum or amorphous solids. The molecular formulas of **4–7** were established as $C_{20}H_{30}O_3$, $C_{20}H_{30}O_4$, $C_{20}H_{30}O_3$, and $C_{20}H_{30}O_3$ based on HRESIMS data, respectively.

The IR spectrum of **4** showed strong absorption band for carbonyl group at 1716 cm^{-1}. The ^{1}H and ^{13}C NMR spectra of **4** (Tables 1 and 2) were similar to those of harzianol A (**3**) [13] except for two major differences: the lack of a methyl group and the presence of an extra hydroxy methylene group. The δ_H signals at 3.41, 3.28, 4.39 (OH) and the δ_C signal at 63.9 suggested that one methyl group was hydroxylated. The ^{1}H-^{1}H COSY cross-peaks between the hydroxy proton and methylene proton, methylene proton and H-5 (δ_H 2.13), along with the HMBC correlations from the hydroxy proton to C-5 (δ_C 40.1) and C-18 (δ_C 63.9), proved the hydroxy group connected to C-18 unambiguously. The molecular framework of **4** was consequently elucidated as harzianol L (Figures 1 and 2). The relative configuration of **4** was determined by ROESY spectra which showed the same correlation patterns as those of **1** (Figure 3). The absolute configuration of **4** was determined as 2R, 5S, 6R, 13S, and 14S by comparison of experimental CD spectrum with its calculated ECD data (Figure 4b).

The IR spectrum of **5** showed strong absorption band for carbonyl group at 1732 cm^{-1}. The NMR spectroscopy data of **5** was almost consistent with those of **4**, except that a methylene group was missing, whereas an extra oxygenated methine group (δ_H 4.21 and δ_C 73.5) was detected. The signals suggested that one methylene group was oxygenated (Tables 1 and 2). ^{1}H-^{1}H COSY correlations between the hydroxy proton and H-8, between H-8 and H-7, confirmed the connection of the hydroxy group to C-8. The structure was then determined as harzianol M by a detailed analysis of 2D NMR data (Figures 1 and 2). In the ROESY spectra, H-8 showed correlations with Me-19, indicating the β configuration of the 8-hydroxy group (Figure 3). The absolute configurations of **5** were established as 2R, 5S, 6R, 8S, 13S, and 14S based on ECD calculation (Figure 4c).

The IR spectrum of **6** showed a strong absorption band for carbonyl group at 1734 cm^{-1}. The NMR spectroscopy spectra of **6** matched well with those of **5**, with just 1 more extra methine group (δ_H 2.26 and δ_C 51.8) and 1 less oxygenated quaternary carbon signal (Tables 1 and 2). ^{1}H-^{1}H COSY correlations between the methine proton and H-3, H-15 suggested the methine group was located at C-3. The molecular framework of **6** was consequently established as harzianol N through a detailed analysis of 2D NMR spectroscopy spectra (Figures 1 and 2). The absolute configurations of **6** were determined as 2S, 5S, 6R, 8S, 13S, and 14S through detailed analysis of ROESY spectra and ECD calculation (Figures 3 and 4d).

The IR spectrum of **7** showed strong absorption band for carbonyl group at 1718 cm^{-1}. The ^{1}H and ^{13}C NMR spectroscopy data of **7** were similar to those reported for harzianol A (**3**) (Table S3) [13], with an extra oxygenated methine group (δ_H 3.65 and δ_C 73.5) and a disappeared methylene group, indicating the oxygenation of the methylene group (Tables 1 and 2). The molecular framework was confirmed as harzianol O (Figures 1 and 2) through a detailed analysis of 2D NMR spectroscopy data, including the key COSY correlation between the methine proton and H-14 (δ_H 2.07), which suggested the hydroxy group connected to C-15. The ROESY correlations between H-15 and Me-19 suggested the β configuration of the 15-hydroxy group (Figure 3). The absolute configurations of **7** were determined as 2S, 5R, 6R, 13S, 14S, and 15R by ECD calculation.

The anti-inflammatory activity of compounds **1–7** was measured by NO production inhibitory assay [20]. The cytotoxicity of these compounds was tested to avoid false-positive results due to cell death, and none of them showed cytotoxicity at the concentrations of 25–100 μM (Figure 6). Hazianol J (**2**), harzianol A (**3**) and harzianol O (**7**) exhibited the strongest NO production inhibitory activity at 100 μM with inhibitory rates at 81.8%, 46.8%, and 50.5%, respectively. The IC$_{50}$ of Hazianol J (**2**) was 66.7 μM, while harzianol L (**4**) and harzianol K (**1**) only showed weak inhibition at the highest concentration of 100 μM (Figure 6). Compounds without "top" hydroxy groups at C-8 and C-18 (**2**,**3**, and **7**) exhibited higher NO production inhibitory activities compared to the compounds with more hydroxy groups (**1**, **4**, **5**, and **6**). These hydroxy groups may reduce the membrane permeability and reduced the activities.

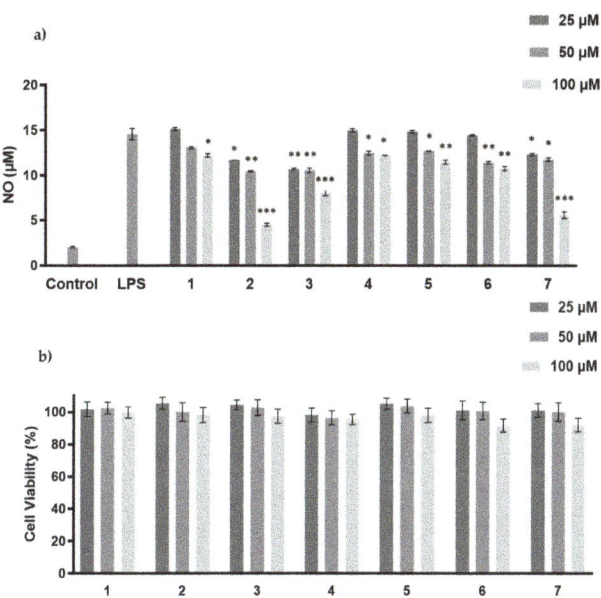

Figure 6. LPS-induced NO production (**a**), and viability (**b**) of RAW 264.7 macrophages by **1–7** treatment. The values represent the mean ± SEM of three independent experiments. *, $p < 0.05$; **, $p < 0.01$; ***, $p < 0.001$ vs. control.

All of the compounds were examined for their activities against plant pathogenic fungi (*Helminthosporium maydis*, *Gibberella sanbinetti*, *Botrytis cinerea* Pers, *Fusarium oxysporum* f. sp. *cucumerinum*, *Penicillium digitatum*). None of the compounds exhibited obvious activities at the test concentration of 100 μg/mL. Since fungi from *Trichoderma* sp. are widely used as bio-control agents, many harziane diterpenes were investigated against plant pathogenic fungi [3,9,10,16,24]. However, the results were controversial. Although harziandione and isoharziandione, the structure of which was latterly revised as harziandione [10], were mentioned as antifungal agents, the activities of the pure compounds were not clarified in the original literature [3,24]. Harzianone was found to be inactive against *Colletotrichum lagenarium* and *Fusarium oxysporum* at 30 μg/disk using a disk diffusion assay [10]. Deoxytrichodermaerin and harzianol A were not active against *Botrytis cinerea*, *Fusarium oxysporum*, *Glomerella cingulata*, and *Phomopsis asparagi* at 40 μg/disk [16]. Harzianone E was not active against *Candida albicans* by traditional broth dilution assay [9]. According to the previous studies and our results, harziane diterpenes did not show anti-fungal activity.

3. Materials and Methods
3.1. General Experimental Procedures

The NMR spectroscopy spectra were obtained on the Bruker ASCEND 600 MHz NMR spectrometer equipped with CryoProbe (Bruker Biospin GmbH, Rheinstetten, Germany). Optical rotations were recorded on an Anton Paar MCP-100 polarimeter (Anton Paar GmbH, Austria), with MeOH as solvent. UV spectra were recorded on a UV-1800 spectrometer (Shimadzu Co., Kyoto, Japan). IR spectra were measured on the Nicolet 6700 spectrometer (Thermo, Madison, WI, USA). CD spectra were measured on a J-815 spectropolarimeter (Jasco Co., Japan). Crystallographic data was collected on an XtaLAB Pro: Kappa single four-circle diffractometer using Cu Kα radiation (Rigaku Co., Tokyo, Japan). HRESIMS spectra data were recorded on a MaXis quadrupole-time-of-flight mass spectrometer (Bruker Biospin GmbH, Rheinstetten, Germany). Normal and reverse phase column chromatography (C. C.) was performed using silica gel (200–300 mesh, Qingdao

Haiyang Chemical, Qingdao, China) and ODS (YMC Co., Ltd., Kyoto, Japan), respectively. Normal and reverse phase thin-layer chromatography (TLC) was conducted using silica gel 60 F_{254} and RP-18 F_{254} (Merck Millipore Co., Darmstadt, Germany). HPLC was performed using Shimadzu LC-16P system (Shimadzu Co., Kyoto, Japan) with YMC-ODS-A C_{18} Column (20 × 250 mm, 5 µm) for separation. Analytical and HPLC grade reagents (Macklin Co., Shanghai, China) were used for isolation procedures.

3.2. Fungal Strain and Fermentation

The fungal strain, which was isolated from the South China deep-sea sediment sample (2134 m depth), was identified as *Trichoderma* sp. SCSIOW21 by ITS sequencing and morphology analysis. Its sequence data was deposited at GenBank (accession number: KC569351.1) and the strain was deposited at the Laboratory of Microbial Natural Products, Shenzhen University, China. The fungal strain was activated on potato dextrose agar dishes containing 3% sea salt at 28 °C for 3 days and cultured in modified rice broth (rice 50.0 g sprayed with 3% sea salt water 60.0 mL for each 500 mL flask) statically at room temperature for 30 days.

3.3. Extraction and Isolation

A total of 100 mL of water saturated BuOH were added in each of the Erlenmeyer flasks which contained fermentation broth. The BuOH extract was collected after 12 h and evaporated under vacuum. The extraction was repeated three times and the total yield was 12.9 g.

The BuOH extract was subjected to a silica gel chromatography with a gradient of CH_2Cl_2-MeOH-Water (100:0:0, 50:1:0, 20:1:0, 10:1:0, 5:1:0.1, 3:1:0.1, 1:1:0.1, and 0:0:100, v/v/v, 2.0 L each) to give 8 fractions (A–H). Fraction B and C were combined and subjected to a medium pressure ODS column with a gradient of MeOH-Water (5:5, 6:4, 7:3, 8:2, and 9:1) to give 5 subfractions. Subfraction 2 was separated by a semi-preparative HPLC column (Acetonitrile (ACN)-Water, 40:60) to give compound **1** (t_R 52.1 min, 9.0 mg). Subfraction 3 was purified by a semi-preparative HPLC (ACN-Water, 47:53) to give compounds **2** (t_R 49.2 min, 3.0 mg), **7** (t_R 32.8 min, 0.8 mg), and **6** (t_R 34.1 min, 0.8 mg). Subfraction 5 was separated by a semi-preparative HPLC (ACN-Water, 70:30) to give compound **3** (t_R 15.9 min, 1.0 mg). Fraction D was subjected to a medium pressure liquid chromatography YMC-ODS-A C_{18} Column with a gradient of MeOH-Water (1:9, 2:8, 3:7, 4:6, 5:5, 6:4, 7:3, 8:2, and 9:1) to give 14 subfractions. Subfraction 7 was purified by a semi-preparative HPLC (ACN-Water, 18:82) to give compound **5** (t_R 29.6 min, 1.6 mg). Subfraction 9 was purified by a semi-preparative HPLC (ACN-Water, 23:77) to give compound **4** (t_R 41.5 min, 1.0 mg).

3.4. Spectral Data of the Compounds

Harzianol K (**1**): colorless crystal; $[\alpha]^{25}_D$ +64.1 (c 0.36, MeOH); UV (MeOH) λ_{max} (log ε) 252 (3.77) nm; ECD (0.12 mg/mL, MeOH) λ_{max} (Δε) 245 (−36.7), 292 (+7.4), 351 (+10.6) nm; IR (KBr) ν_{max} 3402 (s), 2927 (m), 1734 (s), 1695 (s), 1190 (m), 1043 (m) cm^{-1}; ^{1}H NMR and ^{13}C NMR spectroscopy data (DMSO-d_6, 600 and 150 MHz), see Tables 1 and 2; HREIMS m/z: 317.2115 [M + H]$^+$ (calcd for $C_{20}H_{29}O_3$, 317.2117).

Harzianol L (**4**): colorless gum; $[\alpha]^{25}_D$ +15.3 (c 0.28, MeOH); UV (MeOH) λ_{max} (log ε) 256 (3.89) nm; ECD (0.14 mg/mL, MeOH) λ_{max} (Δε) 247 (−36.7), 349 (+2.7) nm; IR (KBr) ν_{max} 3371(s), 2922 (m), 1716 (s), 1653 (m), 1149 (m), 1056 (m) cm^{-1}; ^{1}H NMR and ^{13}C NMR spectroscopy data (DMSO-d_6, 600 and 150 MHz), see Tables 1 and 2; HREIMS m/z: 319.2278 [M + H]$^+$ (calcd for $C_{20}H_{31}O_3$, 319.2273).

Harzianol M (**5**): colorless gum; $[\alpha]^{25}_D$ +14.1 (c 0.15, MeOH); UV (MeOH) λ_{max} (log ε) 251 (4.07) nm; ECD (0.15 mg/mL, MeOH) λ_{max} (Δε) 245 (−8.2), 358 (+4.8) nm; IR (KBr) ν_{max} 3360 (s), 2922 (m), 1732 (s), 1668 (m), 1122 (m), 1024 (m) cm^{-1}; ^{1}H NMR and ^{13}C NMR spectroscopy data (DMSO-d_6, 600 and 150 MHz), see Tables 1 and 2; HREIMS m/z: 335.2229 [M + H]$^+$ (calcd for $C_{20}H_{31}O_4$, 335.2222).

Harzianol N (**6**): amorphous solid; $[\alpha]^{25}_D$ +10.1 (c 0.18, MeOH); UV (MeOH) λ_{max} (log ε) 252 (4.19) nm; ECD (0.18 mg/mL, MeOH) λ_{max} (Δε) 220 (+1.7), 245 (−4.9), 353 (+2.4) nm; IR (KBr) ν_{max} 3379 (s), 2924 (m), 1734 (s), 1647 (m), 1153 (m), 1049 (m) cm^{-1}; ^{1}H NMR and ^{13}C NMR spectroscopy data (DMSO-d_6, 600 and 150 MHz), see Tables 1 and 2; HREIMS m/z: 341.2089 [M + Na]$^+$ (calcd for $C_{20}H_{30}NaO_3$, 341.2093).

Harzianol O (**7**): amorphous solid; $[\alpha]^{25}_D$ +12.0 (c 0.14, MeOH); UV (MeOH) λ_{max} (log ε) 256 (4.11) nm; ECD (0.14 mg/mL, MeOH) λ_{max} (Δε) 255 (−1.8), 340 (+1.1) nm; IR (KBr) ν_{max} 3360 (s), 2922 (m), 1718 (s), 1660 (m), 1147 (m), 1058 (m) cm^{-1}; ^{1}H NMR and ^{13}C NMR spectroscopy data (DMSO-d_6, 600 and 150 MHz), see Tables 1 and 2; HREIMS m/z: 319.2269 [M + H]$^+$ (calcd for $C_{20}H_{31}O_3$, 319.2273).

3.5. X-ray Crystal Analysis of Compounds **1** and **2**

The crystals of compounds **1** and **2** were obtained from concentrated MeOH solutions and 1 suitable crystal for each compound was selected. The crystals were scanned using Cu Kα radiation (λ = 1.54184 Å) on the XtaLAB AFC12 (RINC) Kappa single diffraction instrument, the structures of which were solved by the Olex2 software, the SHELXT [25], and the SHELXL [26] package with the parameters corrected by the least-squares minimization method.

The single-crystal data has been submitted to the Cambridge Crystallographic Data Centre database, with CCDC 2093540 for **1** and CCDC 2093541 for **2**. The data can be downloaded for free from the website http://www.ccdc.cam.ac.uk/ (accessed on 7 November 2021).

X-ray crystal data of **1**: $C_{20}H_{28}O_3$ (M = 316.42 g/mol): monoclinic, space group $P2_1$ (no. 4), a = 8.73030 (10) Å, b = 11.43810 (10) Å, c = 8.99520 (10) Å, β = 110.2970 (10)°, V = 842.468 (16) Å^3, Z = 2, T = 100.01 (10) K, μ (Cu Kα) = 0.648 mm^{-1}, Dcalc = 1.247 g/cm^3, 8392 reflections measured (10.486° ≤ 2θ ≤ 148.666°), 3306 unique (R_{int} = 0.0193, R_{sigma} = 0.0222) which were used in all calculations. The final R_1 was 0.0273 [I > 2σ(I)] and wR_2 was 0.0705 (all data), Flack parameter 0.04 (5).

X-ray crystal data of **2**: $C_{40}H_{60}O_4$ (M = 604.88 g/mol): monoclinic, space group $P2_1$ (no. 4), a = 7.84120 (10) Å, b = 9.31180 (10) Å, c = 23.1108 (2) Å, β = 93.9960 (10)°, V = 1683.35 (3) Å^3, Z = 2, T = 100.01(10) K, μ(Cu Kα) = 0.576 mm^{-1}, Dcalc = 1.193 g/cm^3, 19,167 reflections measured (7.67° ≤ 2θ ≤ 148.826°), 6578 unique (R_{int} = 0.0295, R_{sigma} = 0.0304) which were used in all calculations. The final R_1 was 0.0343 [I > 2σ(I)] and wR_2 was 0.0890 (all data), Flack parameter 0.03 (9).

3.6. ECD Computational Methods

The conformations of compounds **1** and **4–7** were searched by Marvin Sketch software (optimization limit = normal, diversity limit = 0.1) ignoring the rotation of methyl and hydroxy groups. Geometric optimization of the molecules in MeOH (Figures S49–S53) was carried out at 6-31G (d, p) level using DFT/B3LYP through Gaussian 09 software [27], within the 3 kcal/mol energy threshold from the global minimum [28]. The ECD curve was simulated based on TD-DFT calculations and drawn with sigma = 0.3 by SpecDis software (version 1.71, Berlin, Germany). The calculated data was also produced by Boltzmann's weighting and magnetization based on experimental values.

3.7. MTT and NO Production Inhibitory Assay

The cytotoxicity and NO production inhibitory activity were examined using RAW 264.7 macrophages, and the detailed methods were reported previously [20].

3.8. Anti-Fungal Activities

The anti-fungal activities were tested on a 96-well plate by mycelial growth inhibitory assay [29], using actidione as the positive control. Five plant pathogenic fungal species (*Helminthosporium maydis*, *Gibberella sanbinetti*, *Botrytis cinerea* Pers, *Fusarium Oxysporum* f.

sp. *cucumerinum*, *Penicillium digitatum*) were donated by CAS Key Laboratory of Tropical Marine Bio-resources and Ecology, Chinese Academy of Sciences.

4. Conclusions

Herein, we reported the isolation, structure elucidation, and biological activities of seven harziane diterpenes, including five new compounds from a deep-sea derived fungus, *Trichoderma* sp. SCSIOW21. The stereo configurations of the new compounds, harzianol K (**1**), harzianol L (**4**), harzianol M (**5**), harzianol N (**6**), and harzianol O (**7**) were characterized by ECD calculations. Hazianol K (**1**) and harzianol J (**2**) were unambiguously determined by X-ray single crystallographic analysis. Hazianol J (**2**), harzianol A (**3**), and harzianol O (**7**) exhibited weak NO production inhibitory activity. All of the compounds did not show any anti-fungal activities.

Supplementary Materials: The following are available online at https://www.mdpi.com/article/10.3390/md19120689/s1, including detailed 1D and 2D NMR data, ECD calculations, HRESIMS spectra for compounds **1–7**, as well as a brief summary of reported literatures about harziane type diterpenes from 1992 to 2021.

Author Contributions: The contributions of the respective authors are as follows: H.L. contributed to fermentation, extraction, structure elucidation, and manuscript preparation; X.L. (Xinyi Liu) contributed to isolation and data acquisition; X.L. (Xiaofan Li) contributed to the evaluation of bioactivities and manuscript revision; Z.H. contributed to manuscript revision; L.W. contributed to the experimental design, manuscript preparation, supervision, and funding acquisition. All authors have read and agreed to the published version of the manuscript.

Funding: This research was financially supported by the National Key Research and Development Project 2019YFC0312501 and 2018YFA0902504; the Science and Technology Project of Shenzhen City, Shenzhen Bureau of Science, Technology, and Information under Grant JCYJ20180305123659726, JCYJ20190808114415068 and by the Interdisciplinary Innovation Team Project of Shenzhen University.

Informed Consent Statement: Not applicable.

Data Availability Statement: Not applicable.

Acknowledgments: The authors thank the Instrumentation Analysis Center of Shenzhen University for the measurement of NMR spectra and MS data. We also thank the Analysis Center, college of life sciences and oceanography, Shenzhen University for the measurement of IR and CD spectra.

Conflicts of Interest: The authors declare no conflict of interest.

References

1. Zain Ul Arifeen, M.; Ma, Y.N.; Xue, Y.R.; Liu, C.H. Deep-sea fungi could be the new arsenal for bioactive molecules. *Mar. Drugs* **2019**, *18*, 9. [CrossRef] [PubMed]
2. Carroll, A.R.; Copp, B.R.; Davis, R.A.; Keyzers, R.A.; Prinsep, M.R. Marine natural products. *Nat. Prod. Rep.* **2021**, *38*, 362–413. [CrossRef]
3. Ghisalberti, E.L.; Hockless, D.C.R.; Rowland, C.; White, A.H. Harziandione, a new class of diterpene from *Trichoderma harzianum*. *J. Nat. Prod.* **1992**, *55*, 1690–1694. [CrossRef]
4. Wang, X.; Jin, X.Y.; Zhou, J.C.; Zhu, R.X.; Qiao, Y.N.; Zhang, J.Z.; Li, Y.; Zhang, C.Y.; Chen, W.; Chang, W.Q.; et al. Terpenoids from the Chinese liverwort *Heteroscyphus coalitus* and their anti-virulence activity against *Candida albicans*. *Phytochemistry* **2020**, *174*, 112324. [CrossRef]
5. Song, Y.P.; Fang, S.T.; Miao, F.P.; Yin, X.L.; Ji, N.Y. Diterpenes and sesquiterpenes from the marine algicolous fungus *Trichoderma harzianum* X-5. *J. Nat. Prod.* **2018**, *81*, 2553–2559. [CrossRef] [PubMed]
6. Song, Y.P.; Liu, X.H.; Shi, Z.Z.; Miao, F.P.; Fang, S.T.; Ji, N.Y. Bisabolane, cyclonerane, and harziane derivatives from the marine-alga-endophytic fungus *Trichoderma asperellum* cf44-2. *Phytochemistry* **2018**, *152*, 45–52. [CrossRef] [PubMed]
7. Song, Y.P.; Miao, F.P.; Liang, X.R.; Yin, X.L.; Ji, N.Y. Harziane and cadinane terpenoids from the alga-endophytic fungus *Trichoderma asperellum* A-YMD-9-2. *Phytochem. Lett.* **2019**, *32*, 38–41. [CrossRef]
8. Li, W.Y.; Liu, Y.; Lin, Y.T.; Liu, Y.C.; Guo, K.; Li, X.N.; Luo, S.H.; Li, S.H. Antibacterial harziane diterpenoids from a fungal symbiont *Trichoderma atroviride* isolated from *Colquhounia coccinea* var. *mollis*. *Phytochemistry* **2020**, *170*, 112198. [CrossRef]

9. Shi, T.; Shao, C.L.; Liu, Y.; Zhao, D.L.; Cao, F.; Fu, X.M.; Yu, J.Y.; Wu, J.S.; Zhang, Z.K.; Wang, C.Y. Terpenoids from the coral-derived fungus *Trichoderma harzianum* (XS-20090075) induced by chemical epigenetic manipulation. *Front. Microbiol.* **2020**, *11*, 572. [CrossRef]
10. Miao, F.P.; Liang, X.R.; Yin, X.L.; Wang, G.; Ji, N.Y. Absolute configurations of unique harziane diterpenes from *Trichoderma* species. *Org. Lett.* **2012**, *14*, 3815–3817. [CrossRef]
11. Adelin, E.; Servy, C.; Martin, M.T.; Arcile, G.; Iorga, B.I.; Retailleau, P.; Bonfill, M.; Ouazzani, J. Bicyclic and tetracyclic diterpenes from a *Trichoderma* symbiont of *Taxus baccata*. *Phytochemistry* **2014**, *97*, 55–61. [CrossRef]
12. Zhang, M.; Liu, J.M.; Zhao, J.L.; Li, N.; Chen, R.D.; Xie, K.B.; Zhang, W.J.; Feng, K.P.; Yan, Z.; Wang, N.; et al. Two new diterpenoids from the endophytic fungus *Trichoderma* sp. Xy24 isolated from mangrove plant *Xylocarpus granatum*. *Chin. Chem. Lett.* **2016**, *27*, 957–960. [CrossRef]
13. Zhang, M.; Liu, J.; Chen, R.; Zhao, J.; Xie, K.; Chen, D.; Feng, K.; Dai, J. Microbial oxidation of harzianone by *Bacillus* sp. IMM-006. *Tetrahedron* **2017**, *73*, 7195–7199. [CrossRef]
14. Zhang, M.; Liu, J.; Chen, R.; Zhao, J.; Xie, K.; Chen, D.; Feng, K.; Dai, J. Two Furanharzianones with 4/7/5/6/5 ring system from microbial transformation of harzianone. *Org. Lett.* **2017**, *19*, 1168–1171. [CrossRef] [PubMed]
15. Zhao, D.L.; Yang, L.J.; Shi, T.; Wang, C.Y.; Shao, C.L.; Wang, C.Y. Potent phytotoxic harziane diterpenes from a soft coral-derived strain of the fungus *Trichoderma harzianum* XS-20090075. *Sci. Rep.* **2019**, *9*, 13345. [CrossRef]
16. Zou, J.X.; Song, Y.P.; Ji, N.Y. Deoxytrichodermaerin, a harziane lactone from the marine algicolous fungus *Trichoderma longibrachiatum* A-WH-20-2. *Nat. Prod. Res.* **2021**, *35*, 216–221. [CrossRef]
17. Zou, J.X.; Song, Y.P.; Zeng, Z.Q.; Ji, N.Y. Proharziane and harziane derivatives from the marine algicolous fungus *Trichoderma asperelloides* RR-dl-6-11. *J. Nat. Prod.* **2021**, *84*, 1414–1419. [CrossRef]
18. Li, X.; Xia, Z.; Tang, J.; Wu, J.; Tong, J.; Li, M.; Ju, J.; Chen, H.; Wang, L. Identification and biological evaluation of secondary metabolites from marine derived fungi-*Aspergillus* sp. SCSIOW3, cultivated in the presence of epigenetic modifying agents. *Molecules* **2017**, *22*, 1302. [CrossRef]
19. Wang, L.; Li, M.; Lin, Y.; Du, S.; Liu, Z.; Ju, J.; Suzuki, H.; Sawada, M.; Umezawa, K. Inhibition of cellular inflammatory mediator production and amelioration of learning deficit in flies by deep sea *Aspergillus*-derived cyclopenin. *J. Antibiot.* **2020**, *73*, 622–629. [CrossRef]
20. Wang, L.; Li, M.; Tang, J.; Li, X. Eremophilane sesquiterpenes from a deep marine-derived fungus, *Aspergillus* sp. SCSIOW2, cultivated in the presence of epigenetic modifying agents. *Molecules* **2016**, *21*, 473. [CrossRef] [PubMed]
21. Wang, L.; Umezawa, K. Cellular signal transductions and their inhibitors derived from deep-sea organisms. *Mar. Drugs.* **2021**, *19*, 205. [CrossRef]
22. Zhou, X.; Fang, P.; Tang, J.; Wu, Z.; Li, X.; Li, S.; Wang, Y.; Liu, G.; He, Z.; Gou, D.; et al. A novel cyclic dipeptide from deep marine-derived fungus *Aspergillus* sp. SCSIOW2. *Nat. Prod. Res.* **2016**, *30*, 52–57. [CrossRef] [PubMed]
23. Lu, X.; He, J.; Wu, Y.; Du, N.; Li, X.; Ju, J.; Hu, Z.; Umezawa, K.; Wang, L. Isolation and characterization of new anti-inflammatory and antioxidant components from deep marine-derived fungus *Myrothecium* sp. Bzo-l062. *Mar. Drugs* **2020**, *18*, 597. [CrossRef]
24. Mannina, L.; Segre, A.L.; Ritieni, A.; Fogliano, V.; Vinale, F.; Randazzo, G.; Maddau, L.; Bottalico, A. A new fungal growth inhibitor from *Trichoderma viride*. *Tetrahedron* **1997**, *53*, 3135–3144. [CrossRef]
25. Sheldrick, G. SHELXT—Integrated space-group and crystal-structure determination. *Acta. Crystallogr. A Found. Adv.* **2015**, *71*, 3–8. [CrossRef]
26. Sheldrick, G. Crystal structure refinement with SHELXL. *Acta. Crystallogr. C Struct. Chem.* **2015**, *71*, 3–8. [CrossRef] [PubMed]
27. Frisch, M.J.T.; Trucks, G.W.; Schlegel, H.B.; Scuseria, G.E.; Robb, M.A.; Cheeseman, J.R.; Scalmani, G.; Barone, V.; Mennucci, B.; Petersson, G.A.; et al. *Gaussian 09 Revision D. 01*; Gaussian Inc.: Wallingford, CT, USA, 2009.
28. Bruhn, T.; Schaumlöffel, A.; Hemberger, Y.; Bringmann, G. SpecDis: Quantifying the comparison of calculated and experimental electronic circular dichroism spectra. *Chirality* **2013**, *25*, 243–249. [CrossRef]
29. Zhai, M.M.; Qi, F.M.; Li, J.; Jiang, C.X.; Hou, Y.; Shi, Y.P.; Di, D.L.; Zhang, J.W.; Wu, Q.X. Isolation of secondary metabolites from the soil-derived fungus *Clonostachys rosea* YRS-06, a biological control agent, and evaluation of antibacterial activity. *J. Agric. Food Chem.* **2016**, *64*, 2298–2306. [CrossRef] [PubMed]

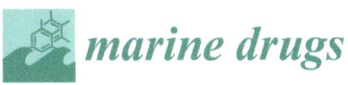

Article

Characteristics of Two Crustins from *Alvinocaris longirostris* in Hydrothermal Vents

Lu-Lu Guo [1], Shao-Lu Wang [1], Fang-Chao Zhu [1], Feng Xue [2] and Li-Sheng He [1,*]

[1] Institute of Deep-Sea Science and Engineering, Chinese Academy of Sciences, Sanya 572000, China; guolulu112@idsse.ac.cn (L.-L.G.); wangshaolu2021@163.com (S.-L.W.); zhufc89@163.com (F.-C.Z.)
[2] Institute of Clinical Pharmacology, Peking University, Beijing 100000, China; xuefeng2378@126.com
* Correspondence: he-lisheng@idsse.ac.cn; Tel.: +86-898-88380060

Abstract: Crustins are widely distributed among different crustacean groups. They are characterized by a whey acidic protein (WAP) domain, and most examined Crustins show activity against Gram-positive bacteria. This study reports two Crustins, Al-crus 3 and Al-crus 7, from hydrothermal vent shrimp, *Alvinocaris longirostris*. Al-crus 3 and Al-crus 7 belong to Crustin Type IIa, with a similarity of about 51% at amino acid level. Antibacterial assays showed that Al-crus 3 mainly displayed activity against Gram-positive bacteria with MIC_{50} values of 10–25 µM. However, Al-crus 7 not only displayed activity against Gram-positive bacteria but also against Gram-negative bacteria Imipenem-resistant *Acinetobacter baumannii*, in a sensitive manner. Notably, in the effective antibacterial spectrum, Methicillin-sensitive *Staphylococcus aureus*, *Escherichia coli* (ESBLs) and Imipenem-resistant *A. baumannii* were drug-resistant pathogens. Narrowing down the sequence to the WAP domain, Al-crusWAP 3 and Al-crusWAP 7 demonstrated antibacterial activities but were weak. Additionally, the effects on bacteria did not significantly change after they were maintained at room temperature for 48 h. This indicated that Al-crus 3 and Al-crus 7 were relatively stable and convenient for transportation. Altogether, this study reported two new Crustins with specific characteristics. In particular, Al-crus 7 inhibited Gram-negative imipenem-resistant *A. baumannii*.

Keywords: crustins; antibacterial peptides; hydrothermal vent; anti-Gram-negative bacteria; Al-crus 3 and Al-crus 7

1. Introduction

Antimicrobial peptides (AMPs) are small molecular polypeptides with antibacterial activity, which is an important part of the innate immune system, especially for invertebrates, due to the lack of a specific immune system mediated by antibodies. Schnapp et al., first isolated an antimicrobial peptide from the blood cells of crab (*Carcinus maenas*) in 1996. This antimicrobial peptide is enriched with proline, with a molecular weight of about 6.5 kDa, and has antibacterial effects on Gram-positive and -negative bacteria [1]. Since then, research on antimicrobial peptides of crustacean has begun. The Crustin family is one of the most studied antimicrobial peptides from crustaceans [2–4].

The Crustin family is largely from crustaceans with a molecular weight of 7–14 kDa and is characterized by a four-disulfide core containing a whey acidic protein (WAP) domain located at the C-terminus, which is associated with multiple potential functions [5–7]. Over 50 Crustin sequences have been reported from various decapods, including crabs, lobsters, shrimp, and crayfish [5]. According to the characteristics of the sequences between the signal peptides and WAP domains, Crustins can be divided into four subtypes as follows. (1) type I: presence of a Cys-rich domain between the signal peptide and WAP domain; this type of antimicrobial peptide is mostly found in crabs, lobsters, and crayfish [8,9]. (2) type II Crustins, mainly found in shrimp, which have a Cys-rich domain and a Gly-rich region of about 40–80 amino acids (aa) adjacent to the signal peptide region [10,11]. They are usually active against Gram-positive bacteria and play a vital role

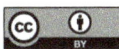

in immune defense for crustaceans [12–14]. There are two sub-groups of type II Crustin (types IIa and IIb), initially classified by differences in the amino acid length of the Gly-rich region and the distance between the Cys-rich region and the WAP domain [15]. (3) Type III Crustins have neither a Gly-rich nor a Cys-rich region. Up to now, they are found only in *Penaeus monodon*, *Fenneropenaeus chinensis*, and *Eriocheir sinensis* [11,16,17]. Many researches do not classify type III Crustin and assign it to the general antimicrobial peptide, similar to Crustins. (4) Type IV Crustins possess two WAP domains and lack a Cys-rich domain [5]. The extra WAP domain at the C-terminal has other potential functions [18–20].

Although the antibacterial activities of Crustins have been widely reported, most are only against Gram-positive bacteria [21]. Only a few Crustins from *F. chinensiss*, spider crab, and *P. monodon* were reported as acting against Gram-negative bacteria with different activities. For example, CruHa1 from spider crab was found to act against Gram-negative bacteria, *Listonella anguillarum*, with a minimum inhibitory concentration (MIC) of 12.5 µM [22]. SpCrus6 from *Scylla Paramamosain* demonstrated weak activity against Gram-negative bacteria, including *Vibrio parahemolyticus*, *Vibrio alginolyticus*, *Vibrio harveyi*, and *Escherichia coli* with MIC >25 µM [2]. Additionally, CruHa1 and SpCrus6 belong to Crustin type I; a type II Crustin, Crus-like Pm, from *Penaeus monodon*, exhibited activity against Gram-negative bacteria with a MIC of 2.5–20 µM [11].

Deep-sea hydrothermal vents are chemosynthetic ecosystems and are extremely hot (200–400 °C), with high pH values and concentrations of heavy metal ions [23]. Due to their unusual chemical and physical features, hydrothermal vents are thought to house unique fauna; more than 600 animal species have been discovered in this extreme environment [24]. Furthermore, organisms living in this extreme environment have unique physiological and metabolic mechanisms to adapt to the extreme environment [25]. Recently, two Crustins, Re-Crustin (type II Crustin) and Crus1 (type I Crustin), were identified from the hydrothermal vent shrimp *Rimicaris exoculata* and *Rimicaris* sp. (Alvinocarididae family), respectively. Although Crus 1 and Re-Crustin shared a low sequence identity (24%) at the amino acid level, they both showed effective activity against Gram-positive bacteria with a MIC of 2.5–40 µM, but no activity against gram-negative bacteria [26,27].

This study characterized two Crustins (Al-crus 3 and Al-crus 7) from another vent shrimp of *Alvinocaris longirostris*. Furthermore, Al-crus 3 and Al-crus 7 were shown to have antibacterial activities on some pathogenic bacteria. Al-crus 7 demonstrated strong activity against imipenem-resistant *Acinetobacter baumannii*, gram-negative drug-resistant bacteria, with MIC_{50} at 12 µM. Thus, this study added new members to the Crustin family and showed that organisms living in extreme environments might contain unique antibacterial resources.

2. Results

2.1. Characteristics of Al-crus 3 and Al-crus 7 Sequences

Two Crustins, named Al-crus 3 and Al-crus 7, were cloned from the cDNA library of *Alvinocaris longirostris* with specific primers designed according to the annotations. The length of Al-crus 3 was 573 bp, with an ORF of 191 amino acids. Al-crus 3 contained a Gly-rich and WAP domain, which are shown by black and red lines, respectively, in Figure 1. The molecular weight (MW) of Al-crus 3 was 20 kDa with a theoretical *p*I of 7.98, which was calculated using ExPasy (https://web.expasy.org/, accessed on 21 September 2021). The length of Al-crus 7 was 702 bp, with an ORF of 234 amino acids. Al-crus 7 also contained Gly-rich and WAP domains (Figure 1). The theoretical *p*I and MW of mature Al-crus 7 were 6.44 and 22 kDa, respectively.

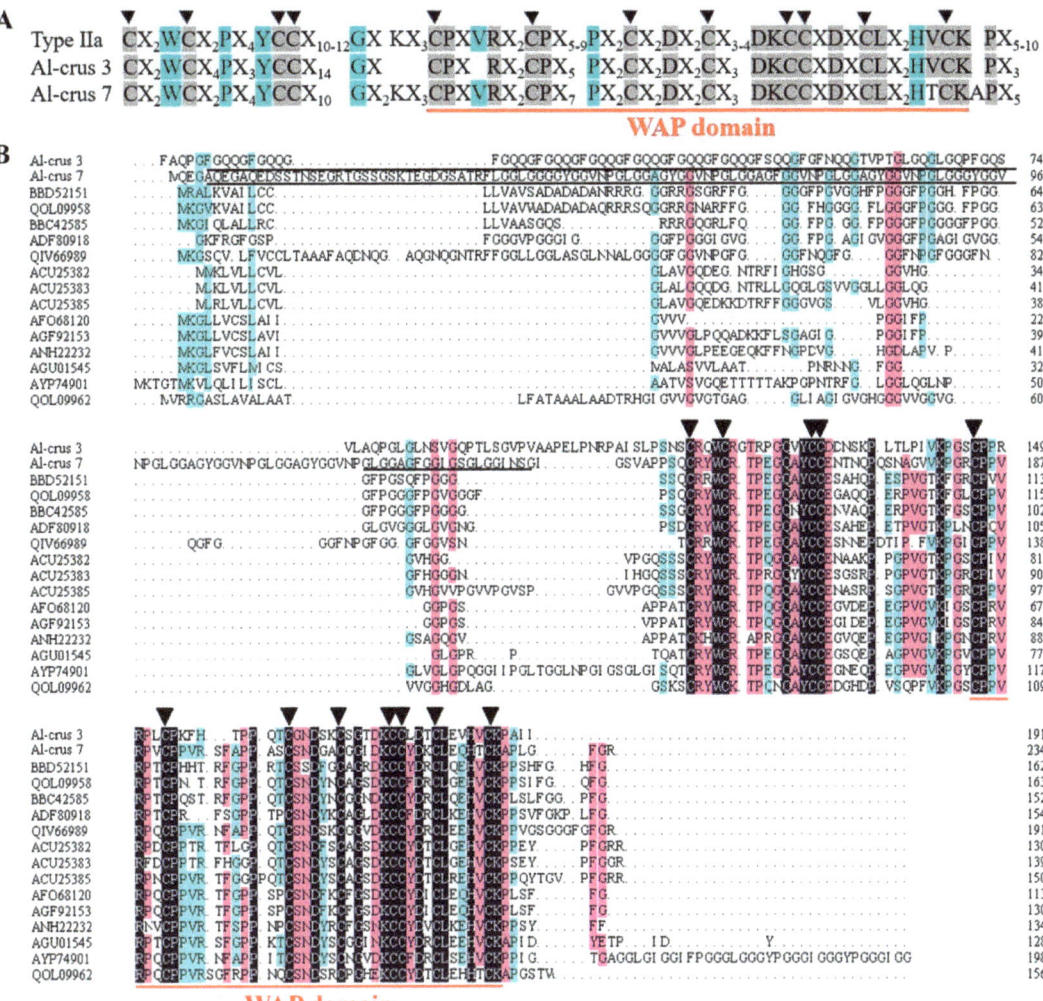

Figure 1. Comparison of amino acid sequences between Al-crus 3, Al-crus 7, and other Crustins. (**A**) Consensus amino acid sequence of Type IIa Crustins. X indicates any amino acid. Identical residues are highlighted. Triangles (▼) indicate the 12 conserved cysteine residues found in the Crustins. (**B**) Amino acid sequence alignments. Besides Al-crus 3 and Al-crus 7, the sequences used in this alignment were from *Penaeus vannamei* (QOL09958, QOL09962), *Panulirus japonicas* (ACU25382, ACU25383, BBC42585, BBD52151, AGU01545), *Macrobrachium rosenbergii* (ACU25385, AFO68120, AGF92153, ANH22232), *Penaeus paulensis* (ADF80918), *Macrobrachium nipponense* (QIV66989), and *Neocaridina heteropoda* (AYP74901). The Gly-rich domain is underlined by a solid black line, and the WAP domain is underlined by a solid red line. Triangles (▼) indicate the 12 conserved cysteine residues found in the Crustins, including the WAP domain.

The deduced amino acid sequences of Al-crus 3 and Al-crus 7 were compared with those of other close Crustins (Figure 1). For Al-crus 3, the closest sequence was Crustin from *Macrobrachium nipponense* (NCBI GenBank accession no. QIV66989), with a similarity of 63% at the amino acid level. By contrast, for Al-crus 7, the closest sequence was a Crustin-like peptide from *Homarus americanus* (NCBI GenBank accession no. KAG7170693) with a similarity of 82% (Table S2). Based on the characteristics of the different Crustin types, Al-crus 3 and Al-crus 7 belonged to type IIa (Figure 1). There were eight conserved cysteine residues in the WAP domain and 12 cysteine residues in the C-terminal region. Among the 12 conserved cysteine residues, there were three amino acids between the first two cysteine residues (Cys_1–Cys_2), a sequence of 16 or 17 amino acids between Cys_4–Cys_5, and a sequence of 8–12 residues between Cys_6–Cys_7 (Figure 1). Thus, Al-crus 3 and Al-crus 7 shared around 51% amino acid sequences. Compared with the other two Crustins of Re-Crustin and Crus1 from other hydrothermal vent shrimps, the identities were 53% and 41% at the amino acid level for Al-crus 3, respectively. For Al-crus 7, the identities were 58% and 47%, respectively.

2.2. Phylogenetic Analysis of Al-crus 3 and Al-crus 7

WAP domain-containing proteins from diverse species were selected from NCBI for phylogenetic tree construction with Al-crus 3 and Al-crus 7. The results showed that these Crustins were mainly divided into two distinct groups: Group I and Group II. Furthermore, there were four clusters for each group (Figure 2); for Group I, the first cluster was shrimp Crustins. The Al-crus 3 and Al-crus 7 examined in this study were also classified into this cluster. Based on the Crustins present here, all the Crustins in this cluster were from shrimp. Some Crustins from shrimp were also classified into other clusters, such as CrusLike*Fc*1 from *Fenneropenaeus chinensis*, classified into the second cluster, Crustin-like peptides. Crus1 from *Rimicaris* sp. was clustered into the cluster of lobster and crayfish Crustins. The fourth cluster in Group I was made up of Carcinins, as they were all from *Carcinus maenas* based on the present Crustins. For Group II, the four clusters were SLPI, SWD, Elafins, and SWAM. The SWAM cluster included mouse single WAP motif protein 1 (SWAM1) and SWAM2 antibacterial proteins.

2.3. Antibacterial Activities of Al-crus 3 and Al-crus 7

The recombinant Al-crus 3 and Al-crus 7 were expressed in *E. coli* BL21 (DE3), and the deduced molecular masses of the two recombinant proteins were 46 and 48 kDa, respectively, including 26 kDa of GST-tag. Seven Gram-positive bacteria and six Gram-negative bacteria were examined in this assay. The results showed that GST-Al-crus 3 mainly acted against Gram-positive bacteria, including *Micrococcus luteus, Bacillus subtilis, Staphylococcus aureus*, methicillin-sensitive *Staphylococcus aureus*, and *Escherichia coli* (ESBLs) with MIC_{50} values of 10–25 µM; whereas GST-Al-crus 3 showed almost no inhibitory activity against *Klebsiella Pneumoniae*, MRSA, and Gram-negative bacteria, up to 50 µM. Compared with GST-Al-crus 3, the recombinant GST-Al-crus 7 demonstrated an antibacterial spectrum that acted against Gram-positive bacteria, *Micrococcus luteus, Bacillus subtilis*, and methicillin-sensitive *Staphylococcus aureus*, and Gram-negative bacteria, imipenem-resistant *Acinetobacter baumannii*. However, GST-Al-crus 7 could barely inhibit the growth of other Gram-negative bacteria. Although GST-Al-crus 3 displayed strong activity against *S. aureus* with MIC_{50} of 10 µM, GST-Al-crus 7 revealed slight inhibitory activity against the growth of *S. aureus* (Table 1). Notably, methicillin-sensitive *S. aureus, E. coli* (ESBLs), and imipenem-resistant *A. baumannii* were drug-resistant pathogens in the effective antibacterial spectrum.

To evaluate the thermal stability of Al-crus 3 and Al-crus 7, the GST-Al-crus 3 and GST-Al-crus 7 were kept at different temperatures for 48 h, and then an antibacterial assay was performed on *S. aureus*. The results showed that there were no significant differences for GST-Al-crus 3 against *S. aureus* after kept at 4, 25, or −80 °C for 48 h, which was also true for GST-Al-crus 7 (Figure 3).

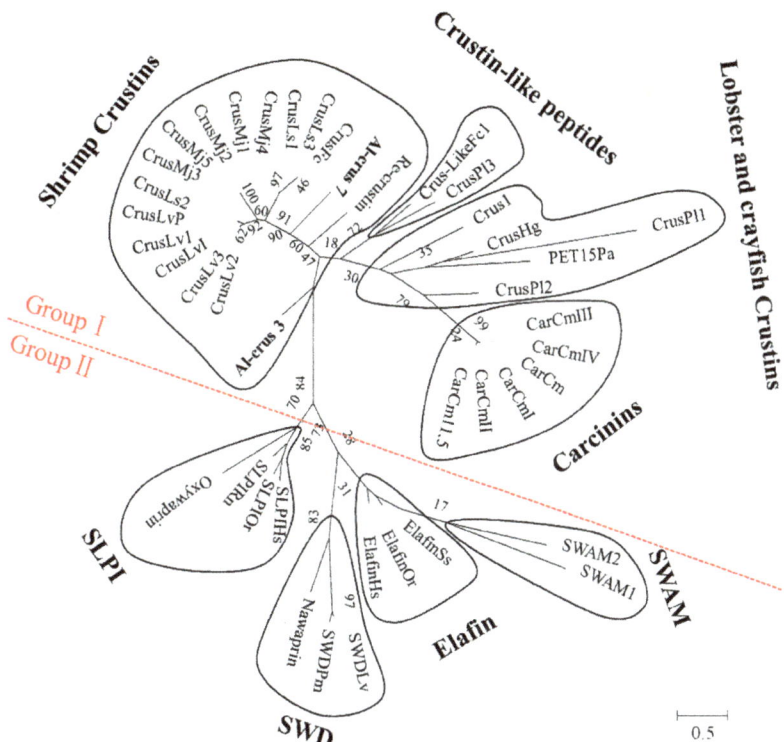

Figure 2. Unrooted phylogenetic tree constructed with Crustins from diverse sources. Crustins used in this analysis from diverse species included *Marsupenaeus japonicus* (Crus*Mj*1:AB121740; Crus*Mj*2: AB121741; Crus*Mj*3: AB121742; Crus*Mj*4: AB121743; Crus*Mj*5: AB121744), *Litopenaeus vannamei* (Crus*Lv*1: AF430071; Crus*Lv*2: AF430072; Crus*Lv*3: AF430073; Crus*Lv*I: AY488492; Crus*Lv*P: AY488494), *L. setiferus* (Crus*Ls*1: AF430077; Crus*Ls*2: AF430078; Crus*Ls*3: AF430079), *Fenneropenaeus chinensis* (CrusLike*Fc*1: DQ097703; Crus*Fc*: AY871268), *Carcinus maenas* (Car*Cm* 11.5: AJ237947; Car*Cm*: AJ427538; Car*Cm*-I: AJ821886; Car*Cm*-II: AJ821887; Car*Cm*-III: AJ821888; Car*Cm*-IV; AJ821889), *Homarus gammarus* (Crus*Hg*: CAH10349), *Pacifastacus leniusculus* (Crus*Pl*1: EF523612; Crus*Pl*2: EF523613; Crus*Pl*3: EF523614), *Panulirus argus* (PET15*Pa*: AAQ15293), *L. vannamei* (SWD*Lv*: AY465833), *P. monodon* (SWD*Pm*: AY464465), *Sus scrofa* (Elafin*Ss*: BAA08854), *Homo sapiens* (Elafin*Hs*: NP 002629), *Ovis aries* (Elafin*Or*: AAQ92320), *H. sapiens* (SLPI*Hs*: EAW75869), *O. aries* (SLPI*Or*: NP 001030302), *Rattus norvegicus* (SLPI*Rn*: AAN32722), *Naja nigricollis* (Nawaprin: P60589), *Oxyuranus microlepidotus* (Omwaprin: P83952), *Mus musculus* (SWAM1: AF276974 and SWAM2: AF276975), *Rimicaris* sp. (Crus 1: MW448473), and *Rimicaris exoculata* (Re-Crustin: MT102281). Values at the nodes indicate the percentage of times occurring in 1000 replications generated by bootstrapping the original deduced protein sequences. Al-crus 3 and Al-crus 7 are in bold.

To further investigate whether the WAP domain is enough for Crustins to act against bacteria, two peptides containing the WAP domain from Al-crus 3 and Al-crus 7, designed as Al-crusWAP 3 and Al-crusWAP 7, were chemically synthesized, respectively. Al-crusWAP 3 displayed the same effect as Al-crus 3 on *Micrococcus luteus* and *Bacillus subtilis*. However, for *Staphylococcus aureus*, methicillin-sensitive *Staphylococcus aureus* and *Escherichia coli* (ESBLs), higher MIC$_{50}$ values were needed compared with that of Al-crus 3. For Al-crusWAP 7, the effects on *Micrococcus luteus* and methicillin-sensitive *Staphylococcus aureus* were the same as Al-crus 7. However, the MIC$_{50}$ of the antibacterial assays on *Bacillus subtilis* and imipenem-resistant *Acinetobacter baumannii* resulted in higher values. These results revealed that although Al-crusWAP 3 and Al-crusWAP 7 demonstrated antibacterial activity, the effect was weaker than that of the full-length of Al-crus 3 and Al-crus 7 (Table 1).

Table 1. Antibacterial activities of Al-crus 3, Al-crus 7, and their deduced WAP domains.

Microorganism	Store No.	MIC_{50} (µM)			
		Al-crus 3	Al-crusWAP 3	Al-crus 7	Al-crusWAP 7
Gram-positive bacteria					
Micrococcus luteus	NRR00100	25	25	10	10
Klebsiella Pneumoniae (ESBLs) *	0244	>50	>50	>50	>50
Bacillus subtilis	NRR00591	25	25	8	25
Staphylococcus aureus	NRR01280	10	25	50	>50
Methicillin-resistant *Staphylococcus aureus* *	H57	>50	>50	>50	>50
Methicillin-sensitive *Staphylococcus aureus* *	G280	10	25	25	25
Escherichia coli (ESBLs) *	G106	25	>50	>50	>50
Gram-negative bacteria					
Escherichia coli (ESBLs) *	K8	>50	>50	>50	>50
Imipenem-sensitive *Pseudomonas aeruginosa* *	E248	>50	>50	>50	>50
Imipenem-resistant *Acinetobacter baumannii* *	E292	>50	>50	12	>50
Imipenem-sensitive *Acinetobacter baumannii* *	H422	>50	>50	>50	>50
Klebsiella Pneumoniae (ESBLs) *	F161	>50	>50	>50	>50
Salmonella sp.	NRR00490	>50	>50	>50	>50

* Means drug-resistant pathogenic bacteria.

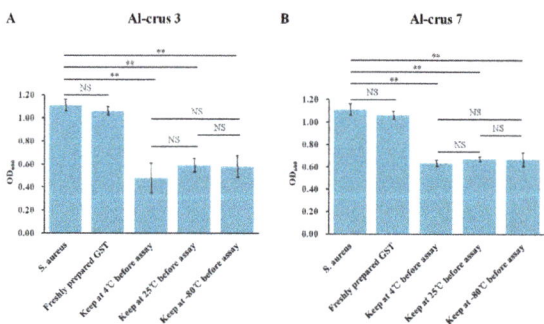

Figure 3. Thermal stabilities of GST-Al-crus 3 and GST-Al-crus 7. (**A**) *S. aureus* was treated with GST-Al-crus 3 for 12 h. Before the antibacterial assay, freshly purified GST-Al-crus 3 was kept at 4, 25, or −80 °C for 48 h, respectively. For control, GST was freshly purified. (**B**) *S. aureus* was incubated with GST-Al-crus 7 for 12 h. Before the antibacterial assay, freshly purified GST-Al-crus 7 was kept at 4, 25, or −80 °C for 48 h. For control, GST was freshly purified. Values are shown as means ± SD (standard deviation; $N \geq 3$). Asterisks show significant differences between Crustin-treated samples and control. **: $p < 0.01$; NS, not significant (one-way ANOVA).

2.4. SEM Imaging

The images of the cells were observed using a SEM apparatus after treatment with GST-Al-crus 3 and GST-Al-crus 7. *S. aureus*, *M. luteus*, and imipenem-resistant *A. baumannii* were used as examples. The results showed that after treatment for 2 h, the cells underwent morphological changes. Specifically, during the treatment of GST-Al-crus 3, the cell membranes of *S. aureus* and *M. luteus* were ruptured and the cell contents leaked; during the treatment of GST-Al-crus 7, the membranes of *S. aureus* became more permeable and the membranes of *M. luteus* became wrinkled. After treatment for 4 h, the number of damaged cells increased. Almost all the examined cells showed morphological changes or were broken after a 6 h treatment (Figure 4). Notably, for *S. aureus* and *M. luteus*, although the cell morphologies changed after treatment with GST-Al-crus 3 and GST-Al-crus 7, their changes were different (Figure 4). By comparison, the cells did not show any change after GST treatment (Figure 4).

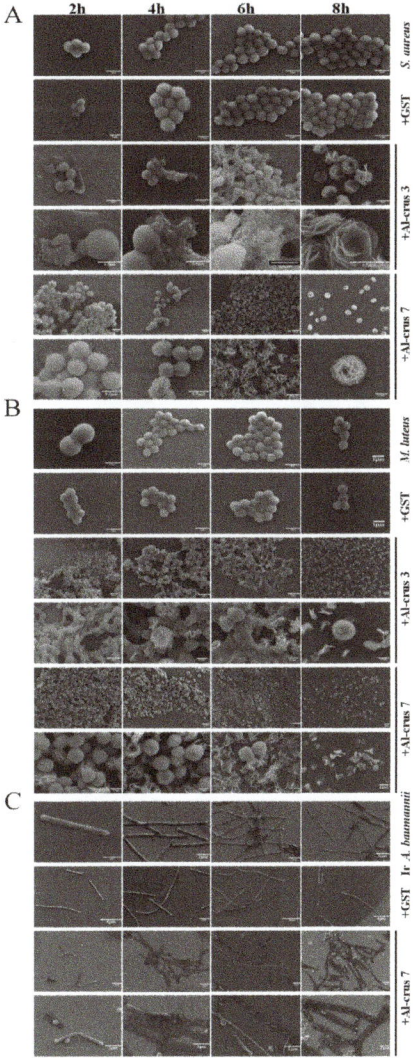

Figure 4. Images of the cells treated with GST-Al-crus 3 and GST-Al-crus 7 at different periods. (**A**) Images of *S. aureus* were observed at 2, 4, 6, and 8 h after treatment with GST-Al-crus 3 and GST-Al-crus 7. GST was used as a control. (**B**) Images of *M. luteus* were observed at 2, 4, 6, and 8 h after treatment with Al-crus 3 and Al-crus 7. GST was used as a control. (**C**) Images of imipenem-resistant *Acinetobacter baumannii* were observed at 2, 4, 6, and 8 h after treatment with Al-crus 7. GST was used as a control. IR: imipenem-resistant.

3. Discussion

Marine organisms are a promising reservoir of bioactive products for drug discovery. Additionally, market analysis forecasts that the global market for marine-derived drugs is expected to reach USD 2745.80 million by 2025 [28]. However, to date, few molecular compounds from marine organisms have been approved and applied in clinics. Furthermore, many marine ecosystems have not been explored, especially extreme environments. Extreme environments feature one or more parameters, such as temperature, salinity, osmolality, UV radiation, pressure, and pH, that show values close to the limit of life. Marine organisms living in extreme environments adopt unique survival strategies for survival and reproduction, biosynthesizing an array of biomolecules that are potentially valuable for many applications, such as biotechnology and pharmaceutics. Hydrothermal vents are extreme environments in the deep sea with high salinity, pressure, and temperature, usually on the ocean floor, such as mid-ocean ridges, where tectonic plates are pulled apart. Although an increasing body of research has been conducted on microbiota from hydrothermal vents, there are few studies on macroorganisms. There is even less research on active molecules derived from hydrothermal vent macroorganisms. For example, there are only two published papers related to Crustins from hydrothermal vent macroorganisms. One study reported that a type I Crustin, Crus1, was identified from a hydrothermal vent shrimp, *Rimicaris* sp. Crus1 shared the highest identity, around 51%, with a type I Crustin from *Penaeus vannamei*. Crus1 demonstrated effective activity against Gram-positive bacteria by binding to the peptidoglycan and lipoteichoic acid of the target cell membrane [26]. Another published study analyzed a type II Crustin (Re-Crustin) from hydrothermal vent *R. exoculata*, which displayed activity against Gram-positive bacteria. In this study, two type IIa Crustins, Al-crus 3 and Al-crus 7, from *Alvinocaris longirostris* were identified and characterized. Al-crus 7 demonstrated activity against some Gram-positive bacteria and one Gram-negative bacterium in this study. Furthermore, Al-crus 3 and Al-crus 7 affected some drug-resistant pathogens. These results reveal the potential of bioactive molecules from hydrothermal vent macroorganisms. The analysis of the phylogenetic tree indicated that the four vent Crustins were classified into different clusters. Crus 1 was classified into lobster and crayfish Crustins and the other three were in shrimp Crustins, although all of the four Crustins were from vent shrimp. Similar phenomena were observed in some other Crustins, such as CrusLikeFc1 and CrusFc; although both from *Fenneropenaeus chinensis*, they were assigned to different clusters. CrusPl1, CrusPl2 and CrusPl3 are from *Pacifastacus leniusculus*, but unlike CrusPl1, CrusPl2, CrusPl3 was assigned to the cluster of Crustin-like peptides. These results suggested that besides the phylogenetic relationships between these macroorganisms, environment microorganisms might be also involved in the evolution of these Crustins.

Antimicrobial peptides are small molecular polypeptides with antibacterial activities that widely exist in organisms, and represent an important part of the body's innate immune system. When pathogenic microorganisms infect the body, they can be synthesized rapidly. When the body produces an inflammatory response, AMPs are generated and released. Furthermore, AMPs are an important molecular barrier for the host to defend against the invasion of pathogenic microorganisms [29]. Antimicrobial peptides have the advantages of low molecular weight, good water solubility, thermal stability, and nontoxicity to the normal cells of higher animals [30]. Moreover, they are easily degraded and cannot easily produce residues. They exhibit different antibacterial mechanisms from antibiotics and can be considered as new anti-bacterial reagents replacing antibiotics. Until now, more than ten antimicrobial peptide families have been found. Furthermore, there are three main AMPs in crustaceans: Penaeidins, Crustins, and anti-lipopolysaccharide factor [2–4]. Antibacterial peptides are highly diverse, except for those derived from highly conserved protein cleavage; different species have specific antimicrobial peptide sequences; even species that are closely related are not exempt. There are seven to dozens of antibacterial peptides in each organism [3,31]. Antibacterial peptides exhibit a broad spectrum of antibacterial activity against Gram-positive and -negative bacteria, fungi, and viruses.

However, the antibacterial spectrum of each antibacterial peptide is different [32]. In this study, two Crustins were characterized. Although Al-crus 3 and Al-crus 7 were from the same species and belonged to type IIa Crustins, they shared a similar sequence of only about 51% at the amino acid level and displayed different antibacterial activities. Al-crus 3 only displayed inhibitory activity against Gram-positive bacteria, but Al-crus 7 displayed it against some Gram-positive bacteria and one Gram-negative bacterium in this study. Even in the activity against -Gram-positive bacteria, their antibacterial spectrum was different. For Al-crus 3, the Gram-positive bacteria against which they acted encompassed *Micrococcus luteus*, *Bacillus subtilis*, *Staphylococcus aureus*, methicillin-sensitive *Staphylococcus aureus*, and *Escherichia coli* (ESBLs). However, Al-crus 7 only inhibited *Micrococcus luteus*, *Bacillus subtilis*, methicillin-sensitive *Staphylococcus aureus*, and *Escherichia coli* (ESBLs). By contrast, Al-crus 7 inhibited imipenem-resistant *Acinetobacter baumannii* with MIC_{50} of 12 µM. The diversity of antimicrobial peptides and their functions are related to the host's response to various pathogenic bacteria and the adjustment of symbiotic flora.

For Crustins, the sequence feature contained at least one WAP domain at their C-terminus. This domain has eight cysteine residues in a conserved arrangement that forms a tightly packed structure, described on PROSITE as a four-disulfide core (4DSC). Previous studies suggest that the antibacterial activity of Crustins is related to the WAP domain. Comparing CruFc with the WAP domain from *Fenneropenaeus chinensis*, which produces strong antibacterial activity against Gram-positive bacteria, CshFc without the WAP domain has almost no antibacterial activity [26]. After mutating the eight Cys residues in the WAP domain of rCrus1 from the deep-sea hydrothermal vent, none of the mutants exhibited bactericidal activity at the minimum bactericidal concentration of rCrus2 [26]. These results supported the viewpoint that the WAP domain is important for the antibacterial activities of Crustins. Nevertheless, no published report has shown whether the WAP domain is enough for Crustins to perform their activities. This study synthesized two peptides, Al-crusWAP 3 and Al-crusWAP 7, derived from Al-crus 3 and Al-crus 7, with only the WAP domain. Apart from *Micrococcus luteus* and *Bacillus subtilis*, Al-crusWAP 3 displayed effects against *Staphylococcus aureus*, methicillin-sensitive *Staphylococcus aureus*, and *Escherichia coli* (ESBLs) with higher MIC_{50} values compared with that of Al-crus 3. Additionally, Al-crusWAP 7 demonstrated the same effects on *Micrococcus luteus* and methicillin-sensitive *Staphylococcus aureus*, compared with Al-crus 7. However, for *Bacillus subtilis* and imipenem-resistant *Acinetobacter baumannii*, Al-crusWAP 7 displayed a higher MIC_{50} value. These results showed that the two peptides exhibited lower antibacterial activities than Al-crus 3 and Al-crus 7, respectively, thus suggesting that other amino acid sequences can contribute together with the WAP domain to the observed antibacterial activity.

4. Materials and Methods

4.1. Strains, Vectors, Reagents, and Enzymes

The bacteria tested in this study, including *Micrococcus luteus* (NRR00100), *Bacillus subtilis* (NRR00591), *Staphylococcus aureus* (NRR01280), and *Salmonella* sp. (NRR00490), were obtained from Huayueyang Biotech Co., Ltd., Beijing, China. The drug-resistant bacteria included the Gram-positive bacteria, *Klebsiella Pneumoniae* (ESBLs, extended spectrum beta-lactamases; Store No. 0244), methicillin-resistant *Staphylococcus aureus* (MRSA; Store No. H57), methicillin-sensitive *Staphylococcus aureus* (Store No. G280), *Escherichia coli* (ESBLs, Store No. G160); and the Gram-negative bacteria, imipenem-sensitive *Pseudomonas aeruginosa* (Store No. E248), imipenem-resistant *Acinetobacter baumannii* (Store No. E292), imipenem-sensitive *Acinetobacter baumannii* (Store No. H422), *Klebsiella Pneumoniae* (ESBLs, Store No. F161), and *Escherichia coli* (ESBLs, Store No. K8). All were obtained from the Institute of Clinical Pharmacology, Peking University, Beijing, China. The aforementioned bacteria were kept at $-80\ °C$ with 20% glycerinum until use. The *E. coli* host strain BL21 (DE3) chemically competent cell was obtained from TransGen Biotech (Beijing, China). Additionally, the vector pGEX-4T-1 was obtained from Qiagen (Hilden, German) and the vector pMD 18-T and Taq DNA polymerase were obtained from Takara (Dalian, China).

The GST-sefinose (TM) resin was obtained from Sangon (Shanghai, China). Finally, the ampicillin, chloramphenicol, and IPTG were purchased from Sigma (Guangzhou, China), the bacterial culture components were obtained from Sigma (Guangzhou, China), and the restriction enzymes were obtained from Takara (Dalian, China).

4.2. Gene Cloning of Al-crus 3 and Al-crus 7

The RNA extraction, sequencing, assembly, and annotation were performed according to our laboratory's published paper [33]. Based on the sequences of the annotated Crustins, two paired primers of Crustins, Al-crus 3 and Al-crus 7, were designed (Table S1). The cDNA library for cloning was synthesized using PrimeScript II 1st Strand cDNA Synthesis kit (Dalian, China). Briefly, a 10 µL reaction containing 1 µL Oligo dT Primer (50 µM), 1 µL dNTP mixture (10 mM), and 5 µg total RNA and RNase-Free dH$_2$O were kept at 65 °C for 5 min, and then immediately cooled on ice. Next, a 20 µL reaction mixture was prepared by combining the following reagents: 10 µL template RNA and primer mixture (from above), 4 µL 5 × PrimeScript Buffer, 20 units RNase inhibitor, 200 units PrimeScript II RTase, and 4.5 µL RNase-free dH$_2$O. After being gently mixed, the reaction mixture was incubated immediately at 42 °C for 45 min and then incubated at 95 °C for 5 min to inactivate the enzymes; this was followed by cooling down on ice. For the targeted Crustin amplification, a 50 µL reaction containing 1 µL of the previously prepared cDNA, 10 µL 5 × PCR buffer, 4 µL of 10 mM dNTPs, 0.5 µL Primer STAR HS DNA Polymerase (Takara, Japan), 32.5 µL ddH$_2$O, and 2 µL of 10 uM for each primer was prepared. The PCR program consisted of an initial step of denaturation at 98 °C for 10 s, followed by 30 cycles of 98 °C for 10 s, 50 °C for 30 s, and 72 °C for 1 min, with a final extension of 10 min at 72 °C. The PCR products were purified and linked into the pMD 18-T vector and transferred into the DH5α competent cells. After being cultured at 37 °C overnight with ampicillin, positive colonies were obtained and identified by sequencing (BGI, Shenzhen, China).

4.3. Sequence Alignment

A Basic Local Alignment Search Tool (BLAST) in NCBI server was used to perform the sequence comparison with the GenBank protein database. The sequences of different WAP domain-containing proteins with high similarity were selected from NCBI and are listed in Supplementary Table S2. The sequence alignment was constructed using ClustalW (v.2.0), and a phylogenetic tree was created using the maximum likelihood model of MEGA (v.6.0) with 1000 replications.

4.4. Plasmids, Expression, and Purification of Al-crus 3 and Al-crus 7

Al-crus 3 and Al-crus 7 were cloned into a pGEX4T-1 vector with the restriction enzymes *Kpn* and *EcorRI*. The procedures of ligation, colony selection, and sequencing were similar to the above mentioned. After the sequence identification, GST-Al-crus 3 and GST-Al-crus 7 were expressed by transferring them into *Escherichia coli* BL21(DE3) cells and then purified by affinity chromatography using GenScript High-Affinity GST Resin, following the manufacturer's protocol (Sangon, Shanghai, China). Briefly, the *E. coli* BL21(DE3) with recombinant plasmid was cultured at 37 °C in lysogeny broth (LB) containing 100 µg/ml ampicillin and 50 µg/ml chloromycetin for 12 h. The cultures were diluted (1:1000) with LB broth and subjected to further incubation until the OD$_{600}$ reached about 0.8, and then induced by isopropyl β-D-thiogalactoside (IPTG) at a final concentration of 0.5 mM. After induction for 12 h at 28 °C, the cells were collected and broken by an ultrasonic binding/wash buffer (1 × PBS with 1% Triton X-100) at 4 °C. After ultrasonication, the cell debris was removed by centrifugation at 8000× g for 30 min, and the supernatant was retained. The recombinant proteins were purified directly from the lysate using GST-sefinose (TM) resin. The supernatant was applied to a Poly-Prep Chromatography Column (BIO-RAD, USA) with 1 ml GST-sefinose (TM) resin, which was pre-washed with a binding/washing buffer. The purified proteins were dialyzed in 1 × PBS at 4 °C for 24 h, with the 1 × PBS replaced every 12 h. The protein concentration was determined using the Bradford method, using BSA (bovine serum albumin) as the standard. The purified proteins were mixed with a 6 × SDS gel-loading buffer, boiled at 100 °C for 10 min, and resolved with 12% sodium dodecyl sulfate-polyacrylamide gel electrophoresis (SDS-PAGE). The gels were stained with Coomassie brilliant blue R250. Finally, the purified proteins were stored at −80 °C in aliquots, unless otherwise specified.

4.5. Peptide Synthesis

The peptides from Al-crus 3 and Al-crus 7 containing the WAP domain were designed and synthesized by GenScript Biological Technology Co., LTD. Al-crusWAP-3 from Al-crus 3: SCPPRRPLCPKFHTPPQTCGNDSKCSGTDKCCLDTCLEVCK, and Al-crusWAP 7 from Al-crus 7: RCPPVRPVCPPVRSFAPPASCSNDGACGGIDKCCYDKCLEQHTCK. The purity of these peptides was more than 98%.

4.6. Antibacterial Activity Assays

The examined bacteria from the −80 °C stock were first inoculated on plates, and then a single colony for culture was picked up in LB broth. To avoid contamination, the tested bacteria were further sequenced and identified. Antimicrobial activities were examined against seven Gram-positive and six Gram-negative bacteria. The MIC was determined by a liquid growth inhibition assay [34]. The purified proteins were consecutively diluted with sterile water in five multiples; next, 0.2% BSA was used as the negative control. Aliquots (10 µL) from each dilution were transferred to a 96-well polypropylene microtiter plate (Corning, Wujiang, China), and each well was inoculated with 100 µL of mid-log bacterial suspension (10^5 CFU/ml) in poor broth (1% tryptone, 0.5% NaCl (w/v), pH 7.5). The experimental assays were grown for 12 h with shaking at 120 rpm/hr and 37 °C. The OD_{600} values were measured every 4 h using a microplate reader (Multiscan FC, Thermo Fisher, American). All the experiments were performed at least three times for the replications. For the thermal stability analysis, the freshly purified proteins were kept at different temperatures for 48 h and then processed to perform antibacterial assays, as mentioned above.

For the peptide antimicrobial activity experiment, the bacteria were the same as those mentioned above. The peptides were centrifuged before dissolution with ddH$_2$O to 550 µM and kept at −80 °C in aliquots. Finally, the MIC_{50} was determined.

4.7. SEM Imaging

The *M. luteus*, *S. aureus*, and imipenem-resistant *Acinetobacter baumannii* were treated with Al-crus 3 and Al-crus 7 with a MIC_{50} concentration, respectively. The treated and controlled samples were collected at 2, 4, 6, and 8 h, respectively. After being washed with PBS, the cells were resuspended in a PBS buffer to about 1×10^6 CFU/ml. Next, the cells were fixed with 4% PFA, 5 µL of which were added to the copper films for incubation overnight. After drying, the cooper film with the cells was examined with SEM (JSM-7100F, JEOL, Beijing, China). The normal and abnormal cells were photographed.

Supplementary Materials: The following are available online at https://www.mdpi.com/article/10.3390/md19110600/s1, Table S1: Primers with restriction enzymes used for cloning, Table S2: The similarities between Al-crus 3, Al-crus 7 and WAP domain-containing protein peptides in crustaceans.

Author Contributions: L.-S.H. and L.-L.G. designed and prepared the manuscript; L.-L.G. and S.-L.W. conducted the experiments; F.-C.Z. prepared and analyzed total RNA sequence; F.X. provided the pathogenic bacteria. All authors have read and agreed to the published version of the manuscript.

Funding: This research was funded by grants from the Institute and Local Government Cooperation Projects of Sanya (2019YD03), the Major Scientific and Technological Projects of Hainan Province (ZDKJ2019011) and the National Key Research and Development Program of China (2018YFC0309804).

Institutional Review Board Statement: Not applicable.

Informed Consent Statement: Not applicable.

Data Availability Statement: The original contribution presented in this study are included in the article/Supplementary Material, further inquiries can be directed to the corresponding author.

Conflicts of Interest: The authors declare no conflict of interest.

References

1. Schnapp, D.; Kemp, G.D.; Smith, V.J. Purification and characterization of a proline-rich antibacterial peptide, with sequence similarity to bactenecin-7, from the haemocytes of the shore crab, Carcinus maenas. *Eur. J. Biochem.* **1996**, *240*, 532–539.
2. Du, Z.Q.; Wang, Y.; Ma, H.Y.; Shen, X.L.; Wang, K.; Du, J.; Yu, X.D.; Fang, W.H.; Li, X.C. A new crustin homologue (SpCrus6) involved in the antimicrobial and antiviral innate immunity in mud crab, Scylla paramamosain. *Fish Shellfish Immun.* **2019**, *84*, 733–743.
3. Jiang, H.S.; Jia, W.M.; Zhao, X.F.; Wang, J.X. Four crustins involved in antibacterial responses in Marsupenaeus japonicus. *Fish Shellfish Immun.* **2015**, *43*, 387–395. [CrossRef]
4. Hoffmann, J.; Schneider, C.; Heinbockel, L.; Brandenburg, K.; Reimer, R.; Gabriel, G. A new class of synthetic anti-lipopolysaccharide peptides inhibits influenza A virus replication by blocking cellular attachment. *Antivir. Res.* **2014**, *104*, 23–33.
5. Smith, V.J.; Fernandes, J.M.O.; Kemp, G.D.; Hauton, C. Crustins: Enigmatic WAP domain-containing antibacterial proteins from crustaceans. *Dev. Comp. Immunol.* **2008**, *32*, 758–772.
6. Hauton, C.; Brockton, V.; Smith, V.J. Cloning of a crustin-like, single whey-acidic-domain, antibacterial peptide from the haemocytes of the European lobster, Homarus gammarus, and its response to infection with bacteria. *Mol. Immunol.* **2006**, *43*, 1490–1496. [CrossRef] [PubMed]
7. Sallenave, J.-M. The role of secretory leukocyte proteinase inhibitor and elafin (elastase-specific inhibitor/skin-derived antileukoprotease) as alarm antiproteinases in inflammatory lung disease. *Respir. Res.* **2000**, *1*, 5. [CrossRef] [PubMed]
8. Brockton, V.; Hammond, J.A.; Smith, V.J. Gene characterisation, isoforms and recombinant expression of carcinin, an antibacterial protein from the shore crab, Carcinus maenas. *Mol. Immunol.* **2007**, *44*, 943–949. [PubMed]
9. Jiravanichpaisal, P.; Lee, S.Y.; Kim, Y.-A.; Andrén, T.; Söderhäll, I. Antibacterial peptides in hemocytes and hematopoietic tissue from freshwater crayfish Pacifastacus leniusculus: Characterization and expression pattern. *Dev. Comp. Immunol.* **2007**, *31*, 441–455. [PubMed]
10. Rosa, R.D.; Bandeira, P.T.; Barracco, M.A. Molecular cloning of crustins from the hemocytes of Brazilian penaeid shrimps. *Fems. Microbiol. Lett.* **2007**, *274*, 287–290. [CrossRef] [PubMed]
11. Amparyup, P.; Kondo, H.; Hirono, I.; Aoki, T.; Tassanakajon, A. Molecular cloning, genomic organization and recombinant expression of a crustin-like antimicrobial peptide from black tiger shrimp Penaeus monodon. *Mol. Immunol.* **2008**, *45*, 1085–1093. [CrossRef] [PubMed]
12. Shockey, J.; O'leary, N.A.; De La Vega, E.; Browdy, C.L.; Baatz, J.E.; Gross, P.S. The role of crustins in Litopenaeus vannamei in response to infection with shrimp pathogens: An in vivo approach. *Dev. Comp. Immunol.* **2009**, *33*, 668–673. [CrossRef] [PubMed]
13. Hipolito, S.G.; Shitara, A.; Kondo, H.; Hirono, I. Role of Marsupenaeus japonicus crustin-like peptide against Vibrio penaeicida and white spot syndrome virus infection. *Dev. Comp. Immunol.* **2014**, *46*, 461–469. [PubMed]
14. Sun, B.; Wang, Z.; Zhu, F. The crustin-like peptide plays opposite role in shrimp immune response to Vibrio alginolyticus and white spot syndrome virus (WSSV) infection. *Fish Shellfish Immun.* **2017**, *66*, 487–496.
15. Tassanakajon, A.; Somboonwiwat, K.; Amparyup, P. Sequence diversity and evolution of antimicrobial peptides in invertebrates. *Dev. Comp. Immunol.* **2015**, *48*, 324–341.
16. Zhang, J.; Li, F.; Wang, Z.; Xiang, J. Cloning and recombinant expression of a crustin-like gene from Chinese shrimp, Fenneropenaeus chinensis. *J. Biotechnol.* **2007**, *127*, 605–614. [CrossRef]
17. Mu, C.K.; Zheng, P.L.; Zhao, J.M.; Wang, L.L.; Qiu, L.M.; Zhang, H.; Gai, Y.C.; Song, L.S. A novel type III crustin (CrusEs2) identified from Chinese mitten crab Eriocheir sinensis. *Fish Shellfish Immun.* **2011**, *31*, 142–147. [CrossRef]
18. Jia, Y.P.; Sun, Y.D.; Wang, Z.H.; Wang, Q.; Wang, X.W.; Zhao, X.F.; Wang, J.X. A single whey acidic protein domain (SWD)-containing peptide from fleshy prawn with antimicrobial and proteinase inhibitory activities. *Aquaculture* **2008**, *284*, 246–259.
19. Supungul, P.; Klinbunga, S.; Pichyangkura, R.; Hirono, I.; Aoki, T.; Tassanakajon, A. Antimicrobial peptides discovered in the black tiger shrimp Penaeus monodon using the EST approach. *Dis. Aquat. Organ.* **2004**, *61*, 123–135.
20. Rojtinnakorn, J.; Hirono, I.; Itami, T.; Takahashi, Y.; Aoki, T. Gene expression in haemocytes of kuruma prawn, Penaeus japonicus, in response to infection with WSSV by EST approach. *Fish Shellfish Immun.* **2002**, *13*, 69–83. [CrossRef]
21. Imjongjirak, C.; Amparyup, P.; Tassanakajon, A.; Sittipraneed, S. Molecular cloning and characterization of crustin from mud crab Scylla paramamosain. *Mol. Biol. Rep.* **2009**, *36*, 841–850.
22. Sperstad, S.V.; Haug, T.; Paulsen, V.; Rode, T.M.; Strandskog, G.; Solem, S.T.; Styrvold, O.B.; Stensvag, K. Characterization of crustins from the hemocytes of the spider crab, Hyas araneus, and the red king crab, Paralithodes camtschaticus. *Dev. Comp. Immunol.* **2009**, *33*, 583–591. [CrossRef]
23. Little, C.T.S.; Vrijenhoek, R.C. Are hydrothermal vent animals living fossils? *Trends Ecol. Evol.* **2003**, *18*, 582–588. [CrossRef]

24. Van Dover, C.L.; German, C.R.; Speer, K.G.; Parson, L.M.; Vrijenhoek, R.C. Marine biology-Evolution and biogeography of deep-sea vent and seep invertebrates. *Science* **2002**, *295*, 1253–1257. [PubMed]
25. Hazel, J.R.; Williams, E.E. The Role of Alterations in Membrane Lipid-Composition in Enabling Physiological Adaptation of Organisms to Their Physical-Environment. *Prog. Lipid. Res.* **1990**, *29*, 167–227.
26. Wang, Y.; Zhang, J.; Sun, Y.; Sun, L. A Crustin from Hydrothermal Vent Shrimp: Antimicrobial Activity and Mechanism. *Mar. Drugs* **2021**, *19*, 176.
27. Bloa, S.L.; Boidin-Wichlacz, C.; Cueff-Gauchard, V.; Rosa, R.D.; Tasiemski, A. Antimicrobial Peptides and Ectosymbiotic Relationships: Involvement of a Novel Type IIa Crustin in the Life Cycle of a Deep-Sea Vent Shrimp. *Front. Immunol.* **2020**, *11*, 1511. [PubMed]
28. Marine Derived Drugs Market Size By Type (Phenol, Steroid, Ether, Peptide), By Source (Algae, Microorganisms, Invertebrates), By Application (Anti-microbial, Anti-viral, Anti-inflammatory, Anti-tumor, Anti-cardiovascular, Other), By Region (North America, Europe, Asia-Pacific, Rest of the World), Market Analysis Report, Forecast 2021–2026. *Pharm. Am. Market Res. Engine* **2021**, 113.
29. Wang, G.S.; Watson, M.W.; Buckheit, R.W. Anti-human immunodeficiency virus type 1 activities of antimicrobial peptides derived from human and bovine cathelicidins. *Antimicrob. Agents Chemother.* **2008**, *52*, 3438–3440. [PubMed]
30. Bulet, P.; Stocklin, R.; Menin, L. Anti-microbial peptides: From invertebrates to vertebrates. *Immunol. Rev.* **2004**, *198*, 169–184.
31. Donpudsa, S.; Visetnan, V.; Supungul, P.; Tang, S.; Tassanakajon, A.; Rimphanitchayakit, V. Type I and type II crustins from Penaeus monodon, genetic variation and antimicrobial activity of the most abundant crustinPm4. *Dev. Comp. Immunol.* **2014**, *47*, 95–103. [CrossRef]
32. Krusong, K.; Poolpipat, P.; Supungul, P.; Tassanakajon, A. A comparative study of antimicrobial properties of crustinPm1 and crustinPm7 from the black tiger shrimp Penaeus monodon. *Dev. Comp. Immunol.* **2012**, *36*, 208–215. [CrossRef] [PubMed]
33. Zhu, F.C.; Sun, J.; Yan, G.Y.; Huang, J.M.; Chen, C.; He, L.S. Insights into the strategy of micro-environmental adaptation: Transcriptomic analysis of two alvinocaridid shrimps at a hydrothermal vent. *PLoS ONE* **2020**, *15*, e0227587. [CrossRef] [PubMed]
34. Roncevic, T.; Cikes-Culic, V.; Maravic, A.; Capanni, F.; Gerdol, M.; Pacor, S.; Tossi, A.; Giulianini, P.G.; Pallavicini, A.; Manfrin, C. Identification and functional characterization of the astacidin family of proline-rich host defence peptides (PcAst) from the red swamp crayfish (Procambarus clarkii, Girard 1852). *Dev. Comp. Immunol.* **2020**, *105*, 103574. [CrossRef] [PubMed]

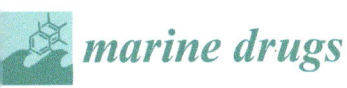

Article

Novel Macrolactams from a Deep-Sea-Derived *Streptomyces* Species

Pei Wang [1,2,†], Dongyang Wang [1,†], Rongxin Zhang [1], Yi Wang [1], Fandong Kong [1,2], Peng Fu [1,3,*] and Weiming Zhu [1,3,*]

1. Key Laboratory of Marine Drugs, Ministry of Education of China, School of Medicine and Pharmacy, Ocean University of China, Qingdao 266003, China; wangpei@itbb.org.cn (P.W.); wangdongyang@stu.ouc.edu.cn (D.W.); zrx1924@stu.ouc.edu.cn (R.Z.); wangyi0213@ouc.edu.cn (Y.W.); kongfandong@itbb.org.cn (F.K.)
2. Hainan Key Laboratory of Research and Development of Natural Product from Li Folk Medicine, Institute of Tropical Bioscience and Biotechnology, Chinese Academy of Tropical Agricultural Sciences, Haikou 571101, China
3. Laboratory for Marine Drugs and Bioproducts, Pilot National Laboratory for Marine Science and Technology (Qingdao), Qingdao 266003, China
* Correspondence: fupeng@ouc.edu.cn (P.F.); weimingzhu@ouc.edu.cn (W.Z.); Tel.: +86-532-82031268 (W.Z.)
† These authors contributed equally to this work.

Abstract: Four polyene macrolactams including the previously reported niizalactam C (**4**), and three new ones, streptolactams A–C (**1**–**3**) with a 26-membered monocyclic, [4,6,20]-fused tricyclic and 11,23-oxygen bridged [14,16]-bicyclic skeletons, respectively, were isolated from the fermentation broth of the deep-sea sediment-derived *Streptomyces* sp. OUCMDZ-3159. Their structures were determined based on spectroscopic analysis, X-ray diffraction analysis, and chemical methods. The abiotic formation of compounds **2** and **4** from compound **1** were confirmed by a series of chemical reactions under heat and light conditions. Compounds **1** and **3** showed a selective antifungal activity against *Candida albicans* ATCC 10231.

Keywords: macrolactam; Deep-Sea-Derived *Streptomyces*; abiotic formation; natural product; antifungal activity

1. Introduction

Macrolactams isolated from actinobacteria have become a large family of natural products, which showed lots of different biological activities and received more and more attention [1–4]. Some molecules with novel macrolactam frameworks and significant activities have been isolated from various actinobacterial strains, such as dracolactams [5], bombyxamycins [6], macrotermycins [7], verticilactam [8], sceliphrolactam [9], tripartilactam [10], and niizalactam C (**4**) [11]. The structure of tripartilactam has been revised to be the same as niizalactam C (**4**) [12]. It possesses a fused [18,6,6]-tricyclic system, which was proposed to be formed from sceliphrolactam via a spontaneous intramolecular [4 + 2] cycloaddition [12].

We have been working on the active metabolites of marine-derived actinobacteria, especially on macrolactams [13–16]. Some interesting natural products with cytotoxic activity, represented by cyclamenols A−F [15,16], have been identified. To further discover new macrolactams for biological study from marine-derived actinobacteria, the deep-sea sediment-derived *Streptomyces* sp. OUCMDZ-3159 was selected. This strain was found to produce streptolactam A (**1**) as the main secondary metabolite. In addition, some trace analogues could be detected by LC-MS. In order to identify these structures, it was fermented on a 30 L scale. As a result, three novel macrolactams, streptolactams A–C (**1**–**3**), together with the reported niizalactam C (**4**) [11] (Figure 1), were isolated and identified. Structurally, streptolactam A (**1**) is a 26-membered cyclic polyene macrolactam [9], while streptolactam B (**2**) possesses a novel [20,4,6]-fused tricyclic skeleton, and streptolactam C (**3**) has an 11,23-oxygen bridged [14,16] bicyclic system. Herein, we reported the isolation, cytotoxic and antimicrobial activity, as well as the complete structural elucidation of compounds **1–4**.

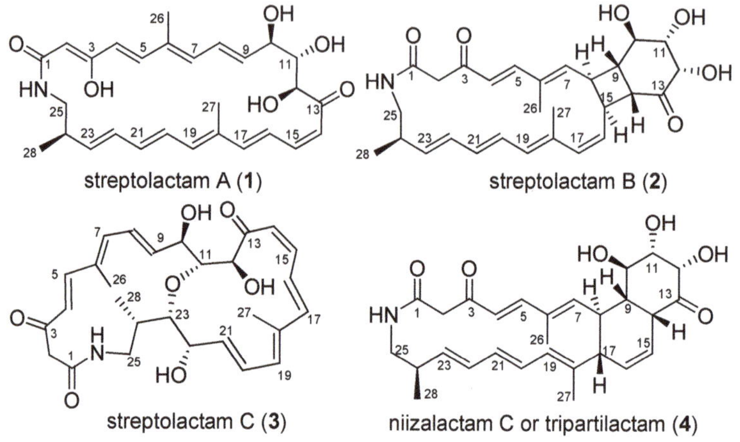

Figure 1. Chemical structures of compounds **1–4**.

2. Results and Discussion

2.1. Structural Elucidation

Compound **1** was obtained as a yellow powder. Its molecular formula could be assigned as $C_{28}H_{35}NO_6$ from the HRESIMS peak at *m/z* 482.2529 [M + H]$^+$ (calcd 482.2537) (Figure S6 in supporting information). The similarity of ^{1}H and ^{13}C NMR data (Table 1) between compound **1** and sceliphrolactam [9] indicated that they share the same constitution, planar structure, which was confirmed by COSY of H-4/H-5, H-7/H-8/H-9/H-10/H-11/H-12, H-14/H-15/H-16/H-17, H-19/H-20/H-21/H-22/H-23/H-24/H$_2$-25/NH, and H-24/H$_3$-28 (Figure 2 and Figure S4), along with the key HMBC of NH to C-1 and C-2, H-2 to C-1, C-3 and C-4, H$_3$-26 to C-5, C-6 and C-7, H-12 and H-15 to C-13, H$_3$-27 to C-17 and C-19, and H-19 to C-17 (Figure 2 and Figure S5). However, absolute configuration of sceliphrolactam was not determined for its extreme sensitivity under light or heat conditions [9]. In the present study, we tried to solve this issue and first tried to elucidate the configuration of C-12 of compound **1** by preparing its acetonide (**1a**) followed by Mosher's method [17] (Figure 2). During the process, the dimethylation derivative (**1b**) of **1a** was obtained (Figure 2). The acetonide **1a** was prepared by treating compound **1** with 2,2-dimethoxypropane (2,2-DMP) and pyridinium *p*-toluenesulfonate (PPTS) in acetone/DMF (3:1) (Figure 2). In the preparation of 3-*O*-methyl derivative of **1a**, we virtually obtained the 2,2-dimethyl derivative (**1b**). However, the $\Delta\delta$ values between *S*-(**1ba**) and *R*-(**1bb**) Mosher esters of **1b** were some inconsistent (Figure 2 and Figures S41–S44), indicating that Mosher's method cannot be used to determine the absolute configuration of this compound. Thus, we tried to elucidate the configuration of compound **1** by X-ray diffraction and luckily obtained the single-crystal of **1a**. A single-crystal X-ray diffraction pattern of **1a** was obtained using the anomalous scattering of Cu Kα radiation, allowing an explicit assignment of its absolute configurations as 10*R*, 11*S*, 12*S*, and 24*R* (Figure 2). Moreover, it should be noted that compound **1** could be isomerized to the corresponding 3-keto tautomer (**1c**) which reached a dynamic equilibrium with its 3-enol tautomer (**1**) in DMSO solution. The ^{1}H and ^{13}C NMR spectra showed some separate signals for **1** and **1c** with the approximate ratio of 3:1 in DMSO-d_6 (Figures S1–S5). The diagnostic methylene signals (CH$_2$-2) in **1c** were observed at $\delta_{H/C}$ (3.17, 3.44/50.8) (Table S2 and Figures S1–S5).

Table 1. ^{1}H (600 MHz) and ^{13}C (150 MHz) NMR Data for Streptolactams A–C (1–3).

No.	1 (in DMSO-d_6)		2 (in Pyridine-d_5) [b]		3 (in DMSO-d_6)	
	δ_C	δ_H, mult. (J in Hz)	δ_C	δ_H, mult. (J in Hz)	δ_C	δ_H, mult. (J in Hz)
1	172.4, C		166.3, C		166.8, C	
2	93.7, CH	4.99, s	50.1, CH$_2$	3.86, d (14.8); 3.65, d (14.8)	50.4, CH$_2$	3.91, overlapped; 3.43, d (17.9)
3	165.8, C		194.8, C		193.3, C	
4	121.6 [a], CH	5.84, d (15.3)	123.4 [a], CH	6.27, d (15.0)	123.0, CH	6.11, d (15.4)
5	138.2, CH	6.54, d (15.3)	149.4, CH	7.28, d (15.0)	146.3, CH	6.74, d (15.4)
6	133.1, C		134.1, C		133.2, C	
7	135.9, CH	5.86, d (10.3)	146.2, CH	6.07, d (10.6)	141.0, CH	6.04, d (11.2)
8	128.4, CH	6.37, dd (13.8, 12.9)	42.6, CH	4.59, "t" like (10.2)	129.7, CH	6.32, dd (14.5, 11.6)
9	136.6, CH	5.43, dd (13.8, 7.8)	50.5, CH	3.52, "t" like (10.6)	139.0, CH	5.45, dd (14.6, 9.2)
10	70.0, CH	4.04, t, (7.8)	70.4, CH	4.40, m	70.0, CH	4.00, t (9.1)
11	74.3 [a], CH	3.79, d, (8.3)	81.8, CH	5.17, m	73.3, CH	3.82, overlapped
12	79.6, CH	4.26, brs	76.6, CH	5.62, m	79.7, CH	4.33, brs
13	199.1, C		213.1, C		198.6 [a], C	
14	119.9, CH	6.24, overlapped	51.8, CH	3.22, m	120.8, CH	6.13, d (11.5)
15	143.5, CH	6.68, t (11.2)	40.6, CH	4.31, m	143.8, CH	6.67, t (11.4)
16	125.6, CH	7.39, t (13.4)	129.6, CH	5.64, m	126.6, CH	7.39, dd (15.0, 11.8)
17	146.4, CH	6.64, d (15.0)	137.9, CH	6.21, d (11.4)	146.9, CH	6.61, d (15.3)
18	134.6 [a], C		136.3, C		136.2, C	
19	135.8, CH	6.24, overlapped	132.9, CH	6.03, d (11.0)	135.1, CH	6.14, d (11.6)
20	135.3 [a], CH	6.18, overlapped	128.0, CH	6.10, dd (14.0, 11.0)	129.2, CH	6.38, dd (14.4, 11.6)
21	127.4, CH	6.20, overlapped	133.7, CH	6.30, dd (14.0, 11.0)	137.6, CH	5.45, dd (14.6, 9.2)
22	131.4, CH	5.81, t (15.2, 9.2)	133.2, CH	5.96, dd (15.0, 11.0)	67.9, CH	3.93, overlapped
23	137.4, CH	5.36, m	137.7, CH	5.42, overlapped	82.4, CH	3.46, dd (8.5, 7.5)
24	39.5 [a], CH	2.20, brs	38.7, CH	2.59, m	38.5, CH	1.83, m
25	43.7, CH$_2$	3.00, m; 3.06, m	46.3, CH$_2$	3.02, m; 3.61, m	50.6, CH$_2$	2.78 d (11.2, 10.9); 3.83, overlapped
26	12.0, CH$_3$	1.80, s	13.0, CH$_3$	1.86, s	12.4, CH$_3$	1.77, s
27	12.0, CH$_3$	1.60, s	16.0, CH$_3$	1.58, s	12.5, CH$_3$	1.61, s
28	16.2, CH$_3$	1.00, d (6.5)	18.1, CH$_3$	0.84, d (5.3)	14.8, CH$_3$	0.99, d (6.4)
-NH		7.73, dd (5.4, 6.1)		8.34, brs		
3-OH		13.69, s				

[a] Assigned from HMBC and HSQC spectra. [b] Measured at 0 °C.

Careful comparison indicated that ^{13}C data of compound 1 (Table 1) were obviously different with those reported for sceliphrolactam [9]. By removal of the calibration of the chemical shifts, we also noted that the most difference is for C-6, C-13 and C-14 which have −1.8, −1.9 and −1.3 ppm difference, respectively. In addition, the value of the specific rotation for compound 1 in the same methanol solution (−392.0 (c 0.05, MeOH)) is different from that of sceliphrolactam (−213 (c 0.09, MeOH)) [9]. Considering no identification of configuration for sceliphrolactam [9], it is reasonable to identify compound 1 as a stereoisomer of sceliphrolactam and a new compound.

Compound 2 was very unstable at room temperature (rt). So, we purified it at a relatively low temperature (18 °C) and measured its NMR spectra at 0 °C. The molecular formula of compound 2 was determined to be $C_{28}H_{35}NO_6$ by HRESIMS (Figure S13). Comparison of its ^{1}H and ^{13}C NMR spectra (Table 1, Figures S7 and S8) with those of compound 4 revealed that they have the similar skeleton. The ^{1}H and ^{13}C NMR data (Table 1), assigned by HSQC (Figure S9), indicated the presence of twelve olefinic carbons, three carbonyl groups (δ_C 166.3 for amide carbonyl signal; δ_C 194.8 and 213.1 for keto carbonyl signals), eight sp^3-methine groups including three oxygenated carbons, two methylene groups, and three methyl groups. Analysis of its COSY correlations of H-8/H-9/H-14/H-15 revealed the presence of a four-membered ring system that was fused with a six-membered ring, which was confirmed by the COSY correlations of H-10/H-11/H-12 and the key HMBC correlations of H-9 to C-10/C-11/C-13, H-12 to C-14, and H-14 to C-13/C-15/C-16 (Figure 3). The fused [20,4,6] tricyclic framework was determined by the key COSY correlations of H-4/H-5, H-7/H-8, H-15/H-16/H-17, H-24/H$_3$-28, and extending from H-19 to H$_2$-25, and the key HMBC correlations of NH to C-1, H-2 to C-1/C-3, H-4 to C-3/C-6, H-5 to C-3/C-7, H$_3$-26 to C-5/C-6/C-7, and H$_3$-27 to C-17/C-18/C-19 (Figure 3). This structure was deduced to form from the intramolecular [2 + 2] cycloaddition of compound 1.

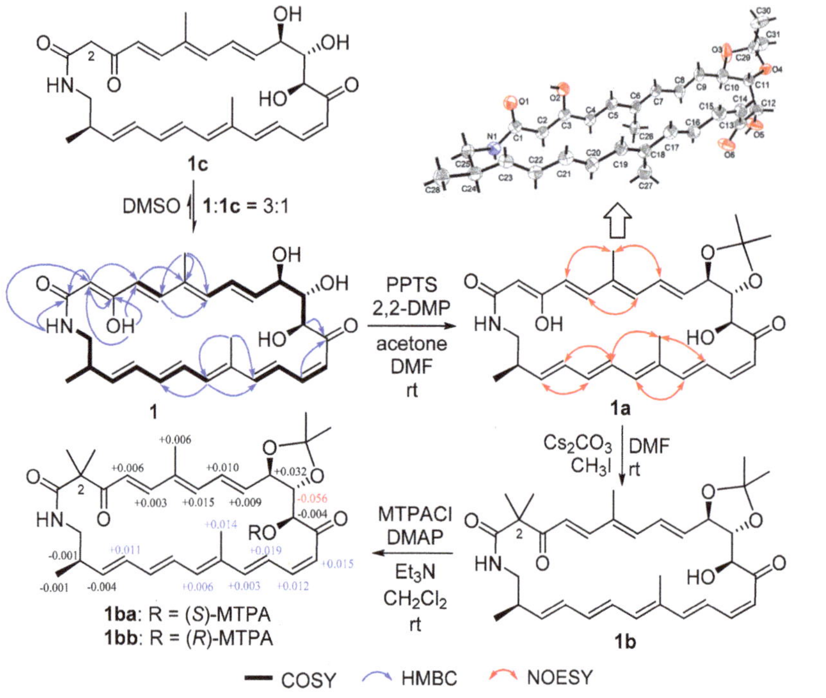

Figure 2. Structural elucidation of compound 1.

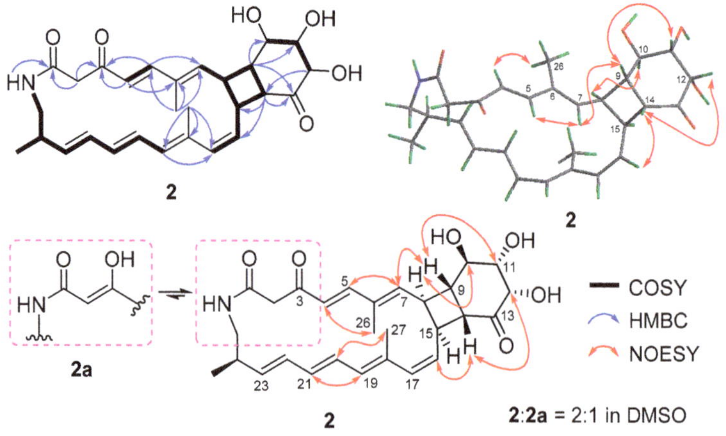

Figure 3. Key 2D NMR correlations of compound 2.

The geometries of double bonds at Δ^4, Δ^{20}, and Δ^{22} were assigned as *E*- by the ortho coupling constants (^3J) of 15.0, 14.0, and 15.0 Hz, while the ^3J value between H-16 and

H-17 (11.4 Hz) indicated the Z-geometry of Δ^{16} double bond (Table 1). The E- geometries of Δ^6 and Δ^{18} double bonds were determined by NOESY correlations of H-5/H-7 and H-20/H$_3$-27 (Figure 3 and Figure S12). The relative configuration of [4,6]-bicyclic system was determined as (8S*,9S*, 10R*,11S*, 12S*,14R*, 15S*)-by the key NOESY correlations of H-7/H-9, H-14/H-16, H-9/H-11, H-12/H-14, and H-8/H-10 (Figure 3 and Figure S12). The fact that compound **2** could be formed from compound **1** (Figure 2) indicated the same (10R,11S,12S,24R)- configurations. Thus, the absolute configuration of compound **2** was determined as shown.

Compound **2**, a 3-keto tautomer, can also be reached a dynamic equilibrium with its 3-enol tautomer (**2a**) in pyridine solution (Figure 3). The ^{1}H and ^{13}C NMR spectra showed some separate signals for **2** and **2a** with the approximate ratio of 2:1 in pyridine-d_5 (Figures S7–S11). The diagnostic NMR signals of sp^2 methine at $\delta_{H/C}$ 5.53/95.3 and enol hydroxyl at δ_H 14.7 in **2a** could be observed (Table S2 and Figures S7–S11). It is interesting that the tautomerization between 3-enol and 3-keto in DMSO or pyridine solution was only observed for compounds **1** and **2**, but not for compounds **3** and **4**. This may be largely due to the size of ring. The 3-enol form could increase the ring tension, so that 3-keto form only exists in the small rings while 3-enol and 3-keto forms can coexist in the larger rings.

Streptolactam B (**3**) was obtained as a yellow powder. Its molecular formula was determined to be C$_{28}$H$_{35}$NO$_7$ by HRESIMS (Figure S20). Comparison of its 1D NMR (Table 1, Figures S14 and S15) with those of compound **1** showed that the signals ($\delta_{C/H}$ 131.4/5.81 and $\delta_{C/H}$ 137.4/5.36) of a double bond in compound **1** were replaced by two oxygenated methine signals ($\delta_{C/H}$ 67.9/3.93 and 82.4/3.46) in compound **3**. The HMBC correlation of H-11 to C-23 (Figure 3, Figures S18 and S19) indicated that the carbons C-11 and C-23 were connected through an oxygen bridge. The COSY correlations extending from H-19 to H$_2$-25 and the key HMBC correlations of H$_2$-2 to C-1/C-3 (Figure 4 and Figure S18) further supported the structural difference between **1** and **3**.

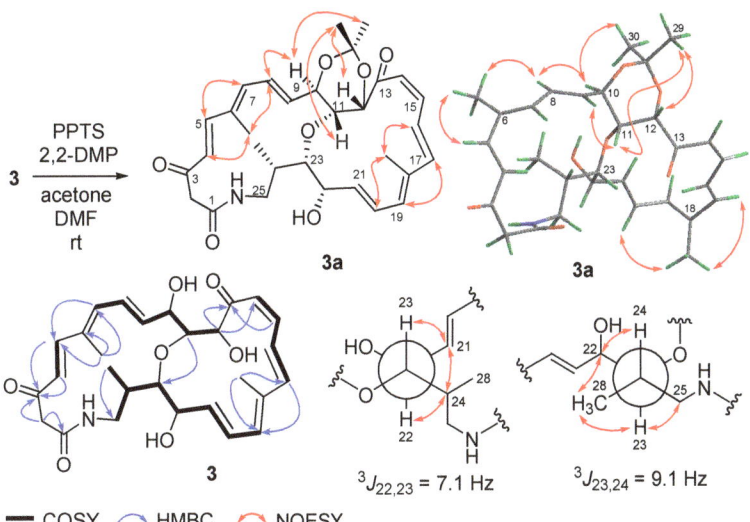

Figure 4. Preparation and determination of relative configuration of **3a**.

The geometries of the Δ^4, Δ^8, Δ^{16}, and Δ^{20} double bonds were determined as E- by the coupling constants of 15.4, 14.5, 14.7, and 14.4 Hz, respectively, while the Δ^{14} double bond was assigned as Z-geometry by the coupling constant of 11.5 Hz (Table 1). In order to verify the relative configuration of compound **3**, the acetonide derivative **3a** was prepared (Figure 4). The correlations of H-8/H$_3$-26 and H-20/H$_3$-27 could be observed in the NOESY spectrum of compound **3a** (Figure 4 and Figure S47), which indicated the E-geometries for the Δ^6 and Δ^{18} double bonds. The (10R^*, 11R^*, 12S^*)- relative configuration was determined by the NOESY correlations of H-9/H$_3$-29, H-9/H-11, H-11/H$_3$-29, H-10/H$_3$-30, and H-12/H$_3$-29 (Figure 4 and Figure S47). *J*-based configuration analysis (JBCA) method [18] was used to determine the relative configuration of C-22/C-23/C-24. The ^{1}H NMR data of **3a** revealed the large coupling constants of H-22/H-23 (*J* = 7.1 Hz) and H-23/H-24 (*J* = 9.1 Hz) (Table 1). The NOESY correlations of H-21/H-23, H-21/H-24, and H-22/H-24 (Figure 4 and Figure S47) indicated *threo*-configuration between C-22 and C-23. The *threo*-configuration between C-23 and C-24 was concluded from the NOESY correlations of H-22/H-24, H-22/H$_3$-28, H-23/H$_3$-28, and H-23/H-25 (Figure 4 and Figure S47). In addition, compounds **1** and **3** might be biosynthetically formed from the same epoxide precursor, **1p**, which subjected to a dihydroxylation of Δ^{22} double bond followed by an etherification between HO-11 and 9,10-epoxide via an intramolecular nucleophilic ring opening reaction (Figure 5). Furthermore, compounds **1** and **3** showed the similar ECD Cotton effects from long wavelength (420 nm) to short wavelength (250 nm), that is negative first and then two positive effects, indicating they shared the same configurations at C-10 and C-12 which were nearest to the two conjugated enone chromophores, C-3–C-9 and C-13–C-21, and thus contributed most to the ECD Cotton effect. The absolute configuration of C-11 could be determined by comparing its relative configuration with C-10 and C-12 in compound **3a**, which is opposite to that of **1**. Thus, the absolute configurations of compound **3** were determined as shown.

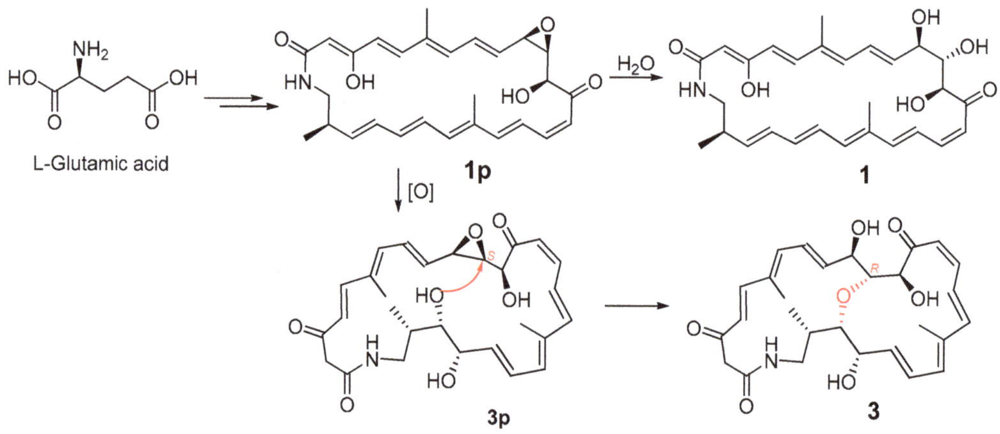

Figure 5. Postulated biosynthesis of compounds **1** and **3**.

Compound **4** was further identical as niizalactam C or tripartilactam by spectroscopic and specific rotation data [10–12]. It is reasonable to strongly suggest that **1** and **4** shared a similar absolute configuration based on the fact that compound **4** could be formed from compound **1**.

During the isolation and structural elucidation of compound **1**, we noticed that compound **1** becomes unstable under light and heat and easy to form compounds **2** and **4**. In order to further understand the transformations among compounds **1**, **2** and **4**, a series of reactions were carried out under different conditions (Figure 6). Compound **1** could exist as a stable structure without light at the temperatures below 30 °C but exhaust and was transformed into compound **4** by the heat Diels-Alder reaction at 50 °C for 6 h, while compound **1** could be transformed into compound **2** via [2 + 2] cycloaddition by light (LED) at low temperature (−15 °C). In the latter reaction, only a little compound **4** was yielded. During the formation of compound **2**, only one product with a specific fusing mode, that is a [20,4,6]-fused tricyclic system, was generated, which might be caused by the geometries of double bonds and their relative position in the macrocycle. When compound **2** was placed at 30 °C, it could be transformed into compound **4**. At the low temperature (−15 °C) with or without light (LED), compound **2** was stable. These results demonstrated that compound **2** might be an important intermediate during the formation of **4** from **1** stored at rt without protection from light. So, light was the key factor causing compound **1** to change at rt. Avoiding light operation is an effective means to keep the polyene macrolactams stable.

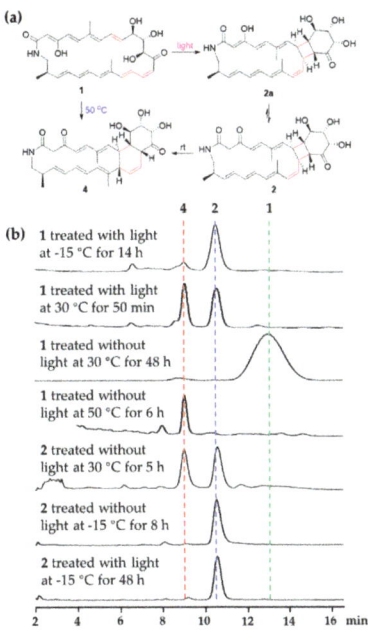

Figure 6. (a) Abiotic formation of compounds **2** and **4** from compound **1**. (b) HPLC profiles (320 nm) of different chemical transformations in MeOH.

2.2. The Bioactivities of Compounds **1–4** from Streptomyces sp. OUCMDZ-3159

Compounds **1**, **3**, and **4** were evaluated for cytotoxicity against MCF-7, A549, K562, and HL-60 cell lines. No prominent cytotoxic activity against these cell lines was observed (IC_{50} > 50 µM). Their antimicrobial activity against pathogenic bacteria, *Escherichia coli* ATCC 11775, *Staphylococcus aureus* ATCC 6538, *Pseudomonas aeruginosa* ATCC10145, *Clostridium perfringens* CGMCC 1.0876 and *Bacillus subtilis* CGMCC 1.3376, as well as the pathogenic fungus, *Candida albicans* ATCC 10231 were also tested without light. It is interesting that only compounds **1** and **3** showed a selective antifungal activity against *C. albicans* with the MIC values of 10.4 and 16.1 µM, respectively. The result of compound **1** further corroborated the reported antifungal activity of the stereoisomer, sceliphrolactam [9]. The biological activity of compound **2** was not tested, because it is very fragile at rt.

3. Materials and Methods

3.1. General Experimental Procedures

Optical rotations were recorded with a JASCO P-1020 digital polarimeter (JASCO Corporation, Tokyo, Japan). UV spectra were recorded on a Beckman DU 640 spectrophotometer (Global Medical Instrumentation, Inc., Ramsey, MN, USA). IR spectra were obtained on a Nicolet Nexus 470 spectrophotometer in KBr discs (Thermo Fisher Scientific, Madison, WI, USA). NMR spectra were recorded on a Bruker Avance 600 spectrometer (Bruker BioSpin AG, Fällanden, Switzerland). ECD spectra were measured on JASCO J-815 spectrometer (JASCO Corporation, Tokyo, Japan). HRESIMS were measured on a Q-TOF Ultima Global GAA076 LC mass spectrometer (Waters Corporation, Milford, MA, USA). Semipreparative

HPLC was performed using an ODS column (YMC-pack ODS-A, 10 × 250 mm, 5 μm, 4.0 mL/min). TLC and column chromatography (CC) were performed on plates pre-coated with silica gel GF254 (10–40 μm) and over silica gel (200–300 mesh, Qingdao Marine Chemical Factory, Qingdao, China), and Sephadex LH-20 (Amersham Biosciences, Uppsala, Sweden), respectively. Vacuum-liquid chromatography (VLC) was carried out over silica gel H (Qingdao Marine Chemical Factory).

3.2. Collection and Phylogenetic Analysis

The actinobacterial strain, *Streptomyces* sp. OUCMDZ-3159, was isolated from a deep-sea sediment collected at depth of 2782 m from the South Mid-Atlantic Ridge (15°9.972′ S, 13°21.348′ W) on October 31, 2012. The sample (2 g) was dried over 24 h in an incubator at 35 °C. The dried sample was diluted to 10^{-3} g/mL, 100 μL of which was dispersed across a solid-phase agar plate (10 g raffinose, 1 g L-histide, 0.5 g $MgSO_4 \cdot 7H_2O$, 0.01 g $FeSO_4 \cdot 7H_2O$, 0.1 g K_2HPO_4, 1.2 g bacto-agar, in 1 L seawater, pH 7.0) and incubated at 28 °C for 10 days. A single colony was transferred to Gause's synthetic agar media. Analysis of the 16S rRNA gene sequence of OUCMDZ-3159 revealed 100% identity to *Streptomyces pratensis*. The sequence is deposited in GenBank under accession no. MT703834.

3.3. Cultivation and Extraction

The spores of *Streptomyces* sp. OUCMDZ-3159 were directly transferred to 150 mL of a liquid medium (20 g glucose, 4 g yeast extract, 2 g peptone, 2 g $CaCO_3$, 0.5 g $MgSO_4$, 0.5 g K_2HPO_4, 0.5 g NH_4SO_4, in 1 L seawater) in Erlenmeyer flasks (500 mL) and shaken for 14 days (28 ± 0.5 °C, 180 rpm). The whole culture (30 L) was extracted with an equal volume of ethyl acetate (EtOAc) for three times and concentrated in vacuo to yield 20.5 g of EtOAc extract.

3.4. Purification

The EtOAc extract (20.5 g) was separated into nine fractions (Fr.1–Fr.9) on a silica gel VLC column using step gradient elution with CH_2Cl_2–petroleum ether (0–50%) and then MeOH–CH_2Cl_2 (0–50%). Fraction 6 was separated into six fractions (Fr.6.1–Fr.6.6) by Sephadex LH-20 eluting with MeOH–CH_2Cl_2 (1:1) without light. Fr.6.3 was purified by semipreparative HPLC on an ODS column using the solvent system of 40% MeOH aqueous solution to yield compound **3** (16.0 mg, t_R 12.5 min). Fr.6.4 was purified by semipreparative HPLC on an ODS column using the solvent system of 65% MeOH aqueous solution to give compounds **4** (5.5 mg, t_R 9.1 min), **2** (1.2 mg, t_R 10.2 min), and **1** (10.1 mg, t_R 12.3 min). Fraction 7 was fractionated into five subfractions (Fr.7.1–Fr.7.5) on a reversed-phase silica gel column, eluting with a step gradient of MeOH–H_2O (10–100%) without light. Fr.7.3 and Fr.7.4 were purified by semipreparative HPLC on an ODS column using the solvent system of 65% MeOH and 40% MeOH aqueous solutions to yield compounds **1** (63 mg, t_R 12.3 min) and **3** (3.0 mg, t_R 12.5 min) without light, respectively.

3.5. Preparation of Compounds **1a** and **3a**

Compound **1** (25.0 mg) was dissolved in the mixture of DMF (6 mL) and acetone (2 mL), and then pyridinium *p*-toluenesulfonate (PPTS, 3.0 mg) and 2,2-dimethoxypropane (DMP, 200 μL) were added at 0 °C. The reaction mixture was stirred for 10 h at rt. Then 5 mL of H_2O was added, and the solution was extracted three times with EtOAc (5 mL for each). The organic layer was combined and evaporated under reduced pressure to give a yellow gum that was subjected to HPLC purification eluting with 75% MeOH aqueous solution to give compound **1a** (15.3 mg, t_R 10.4 min, 56% yield). The same reaction of compound **3** (5.0 mg) was carried out and the product **3a** (2.0 mg, t_R 12.5 min, 37% yield) was purified by HPLC on an ODS column using 55% MeOH aqueous solution.

3.6. Preparation of Compound 1b

Compound **1a** (5.0 mg) was dissolved in 1 mL of dimethylformamide (DMF), then Cs_2CO_3 (2.0 mg) and CH_3I (1 µL) were added at 0 °C. The reaction mixture was stirred for 2 h at 28 °C. Then 2 mL of H_2O was added, and the solution was extracted three times with ethyl acetate (5 mL for each). The organic layer was combined and evaporated under reduced pressure to give a yellow gum that was purified by HPLC eluting with 80% MeOH aqueous solution to yield compound **1b** (2.0 mg, t_R 7.9 min, 38% yield).

3.7. Preparation of S-MTPA Ester (1ba) and R-MTPA Ester (1bb) of Compound 1b

Compound **1b** (1.0 mg) was dissolved in CH_2Cl_2 (1 mL), and then triethylamine (10 µL), dimethylaminopyridine (DMAP, 3.0 mg) and (*R*)-MTPACl (10 µL) were added. The reaction mixture was stirred for 6 h at rt. Then 1 mL of H_2O was added, and the solution was extracted three times with CH_2Cl_2 (5 mL for each). The residue after removal of CH_2Cl_2 under reduced pressure was purified by semipreparative HPLC (90% MeOH) to yield (*S*)-MTPA ester **1ba** (1.0 mg, t_R 9.02 min). With the same method, (*R*)-MTPA ester **1bb** (1.0 mg, t_R 8.54 min) was obtained from the reaction of **1b** (1.0 mg) with (*S*)-MTPACl.

3.8. Characterization of the Compounds

Streptolactam A (**1**): yellow powder; $[\alpha]_D^{25}$ −392.0 (*c* 0.05, MeOH); ECD (1.00 *mM*, MeOH) λ_{max} ($\Delta\varepsilon$) 216 (−8.8), 281 (+12.6), 330 (+4.0), 418 (−6.7) nm; UV (MeOH) λ_{max} (log ε) 279 (3.20), 332 (3.39), 421 (2.77) nm; IR (KBr) ν_{max} 3549, 3474, 3415, 3239, 2925, 2853, 1637, 1618, 1571, 1427, 1385, 1058, 619, 477 cm^{-1}; ^1H and ^{13}C NMR, see Table S1; HRESIMS *m/z* 482.2529 $[M + H]^+$ (calcd for $C_{28}H_{36}NO_6$, 482.2537).

Streptolactam B (**2**): yellowed powder; ^1H and ^{13}C NMR at 0 °C, see Table 1; HRESIMS *m/z* 482.2548 $[M + H]^+$ (calcd for $C_{28}H_{36}NO_6$, 482.2537).

Streptolactam C (**3**): yellow solid; $[\alpha]_D^{15}$ −792.9 (*c* 0.05, MeOH); ECD (0.10 *mM*, MeOH) λ_{max} ($\Delta\varepsilon$) 256 (+18.8), 319 (+4.1), 394 (−12.3) nm; UV (MeOH) λ_{max} (log ε) 401 (4.92), 319 (4.92), 296 (4.90) nm; IR (KBr) ν_{max} 3357, 2961, 2922, 1680, 1618, 1589, 1455, 1384, 1329, 1263, 1089, 1056, 976 cm^{-1}; ^1H and ^{13}C NMR, see Table 1; HRESIMS *m/z* 498.2491 $[M + H]^+$ (calcd for $C_{28}H_{36}NO_7$, 498.2486).

Niizalactam C or Tripartilactam (**4**): yellow powder; $[\alpha]_D^{25}$ +30.0 (*c* 0.1, DMSO), −75.0 (*c* 0.1, MeOH); ECD (1.04 *mM*, MeOH) λ_{max} 201 (+5.24), 296 (−7.2) nm; ^1H and ^{13}C NMR, see Table S1; HRESIMS *m/z* 482.2544 $[M + H]^+$ (calcd for $C_{28}H_{36}NO_6$, 482.2537).

Compound **1a**: orange solid; ^1H and ^{13}C NMR, see Table S2; HRESIMS *m/z* 522.2864 $[M + H]^+$ (calcd for $C_{31}H_{40}NO_6$, 522.2850).

Compound **1b**: orange solid; ^1H and ^{13}C NMR, see Table S2; HRESIMS *m/z* 550.3167 $[M + H]^+$ (calcd for $C_{33}H_{44}NO_6$, 550.3163).

Compound **3a**: yellow solid; ^1H NMR (600 MHz, DMSO-d_6): δ 7.17 (1H, dd, *J* = 15.5, 11.5 Hz, H-16), 6.77 (1H, d, *J* = 15.5 Hz, H-5), 6.61 (1H, t, *J* = 11.5 Hz, H-15), 6.60 (1H, d, *J* = 15.5 Hz, H-17), 6.49 (1H, dd, *J* = 14.8, 11.5 Hz, H-8), 6.41 (1H, dd, *J* = 14.3, 11.5 Hz, H-20), 6.21 (1H, d, *J* = 11.5 Hz, H-14), 6.14 (1H, d, *J* = 15.5 Hz, H-4), 6.13 (1H, d, *J* = 14.8 Hz, H-7), 6.12 (1H, d, *J* = 11.5 Hz, H-19), 5.52 (1H, dd, *J* = 14.7, 9.0 Hz, H-9), 5.46 (1H, dd, *J* = 15.0, 10.3 Hz, H-21), 4.64 (1H, d, *J* = 1.8 Hz, H-12), 4.37 (1H, d, *J* = 9.0 Hz, H-10), 4.15 (1H, dd, *J* = 9.0, 1.8 Hz, H-11), 3.91 (1H, d, *J* = 18.1 Hz, H-2a), 3.88 (1H, dd, *J* = 10.3, 7.1 Hz, H-22), 3.86 (1H, dd, *J* = 11.2, 7.7 Hz, H-25a), 3.47 (1H, d, *J* = 18.1 Hz, H-2b), 3.44 (1H, dd, *J* = 9.1, 7.1 Hz, H-23), 2.77 (1H, t, *J* = 11.2 Hz, H-25b), 1.85 (1H, m, H-24), 1.81 (3H, s, CH_3-26), 1.61 (3H, s, CH_3-27), 1.01 (3H, d, *J* = 6.7 Hz, CH_3-28), 1.33 (3H, s, CH_3-29), 1.35 (3H, s, CH_3-30); HRESIMS *m/z* 538.2809 $[M + H]^+$ (calcd for $C_{31}H_{40}NO_7$, 538.2799), 560.2628 $[M + Na]^+$ (calcd for $C_{31}H_{39}NO_7Na$, 560.2619).

S-MTPA ester (**1ba**) of **1b**: ^1H NMR (600 MHz, $CDCl_3$): δ 7.58 (1H, m, NH), 7.31 (1H, dd, *J* = 15.5, 12.0 Hz, H-16), 7.02 (1H, d, *J* = 14.8 Hz, H-4), 6.66 (1H, t, *J* = 11.5 Hz, H-15), 6.61 (1H, d, *J* = 15.1 Hz, H-17), 6.59 (1H, dd, *J* = 14.3, 11.4 Hz, H-8&21), 6.54 (1H, d, *J* = 15.1 Hz, H-5), 6.33 (1H, d, *J* = 12.5 Hz, H-19), 6.06 (1H, overlapped, H-7&14), 6.04 (2H, overlapped, H-20&22), 5.73 (1H, d, *J* = 2.3 Hz, H-12), 5.46 (1H, overlapped, H-9), 5.44 (1H, overlapped, H-23), 4.54 (1H, t, *J* = 8.1 Hz, H-10), 4.16 (1H, dd, *J* = 8.4, 2.3 Hz, H-11), 3.66 (1H, dd, J = 8.0, 4.6 Hz, H-25a), 2.60 (1H, ddd, J = 13.0, 10.7, 3.9 Hz, H-25b), 2.51 (1H, m, H-24), 1.87 (3H, s, H-26), 1.79 (3H, s, H$_3$-27), 1.54 (3H, s), 1.42 (3H, s), 1.34 (3H, s), 1.05 (1H, d, J = 6.6 Hz, H$_3$-28), 1.02 (3H, s); ESIMS m/z 766.5 [M + H]$^+$.

R-MTPA ester (**1bb**) of **1b**: ^{1}H NMR (600 MHz, CDCl$_3$): δ 7.57 (1H, m, NH), 7.29 (1H, dd, J = 14.9, 11.0 Hz, H-16), 7.02 (1H, d, J = 15.1 Hz, H-4), 6.65 (1H, t, J = 11.2 Hz, H-15), 6.60 (1H, d, J = 15.0 Hz, H-17), 6.56 (1H, overlapped, H-8&21), 6.53 (1H, d, J = 14.9 Hz, H-5), 6.33 (1H, d, J = 11.3 Hz, H-19), 6.05 (1H, overlapped, H-7&14), 6.03 (2H, overlapped, H-20&22), 5.74 (1H, d, J = 2.2 Hz, H-12), 5.46 (1H, overlapped, H-9), 5.44 (1H, overlapped, H-23), 4.51 (1H, t, J = 8.1 Hz, H-10), 4.22 (1H, dd, J = 8.5, 2.2 Hz, H-11), 3.66 (1H, m, H-25a), 2.61 (1H, ddd, J = 18.2, 14.4, 4.0 Hz, H-25b), 2.51 (1H, m, H-24), 1.87 (3H, s, H$_3$-26), 1.77 (3H, s, H$_3$-27), 1.54 (3H, s), 1.43 (3H, s), 1.42 (3H, s), 1.35 (3H, s), 1.05 (1H, d, J = 6.6 Hz, H$_3$-28); ESIMS m/z 766.4 [M + H]$^+$.

3.9. X-ray Crystallographic Analysis

Compound **1a** was obtained as an orange crystal with molecular formula of C$_{31}$H$_{39}$NO$_6$ from CH$_2$Cl$_2$/MeOH. Further, the crystal data were got on a Bruker Smart APEXDUO area detector diffractometer with graphite monochromated Cu-Kα radiation (λ = 1.54178 Å) (Table S4). The structure was solved by direct methods (SHELXS-97) and expanded using Fourier techniques (SHELXL-97). Crystallographic data (excluding structure factors) for structure **1a** in this paper have been deposited in the Cambridge Crystallographic Data Centre as supplementary publication number CCDC 996760.

*3.10. Chemical Interconversion of Compounds **1**, **2** and **4***

Streptolactam A (**1**), isolated from an EtOAc extract from *Streptomyces* sp. OUCMDZ-3159 without light, was dissolved in MeOH at a concentration of 2.5 mM and stirred with or without light at rt (30 °C), −15 °C and 50 °C, respectively. Compound **2** was dissolved in MeOH at a concentration of 1 mM with or without light at rt (30 °C) and −15 °C, respectively. The reaction mixtures were analyzed every 30 min by use of HPLC on an ODS column eluting with 65% MeOH aqueous solution at a flow rate of 1 mL/min. The isolated compounds **1**, **2** and **4** were used as the standards (Figure 6).

Compound **2** was very fragile at rt. In order to identify its structure, we tried to obtain more materials through chemical transformation. Compound **1** was not stable under light, which could be converted into compounds **2** and **4**. So, we treated compound **1** (35.0 mg, 25 mM in MeOH) with sunlight for 1.5 h, and then the mixture was separated by HPLC on an ODS column at 18 °C using 65% MeOH aqueous solution to yield compounds **4** (4.0 mg, t_R 9.1 min, 11.4% yield) and **2** (2.0 mg, t_R 10.2 min, 5.7% yield). The NMR spectra of compound **2** were measured at 0 °C in pyridine-d_5.

3.11. Cytotoxicity Assay

Cytotoxicity was assayed against A549 and MCF-7 cell lines by the MTT [19], and K562 and HL-60 cell lines CCK-8 [20] methods. Adriamycin was used as the positive control with the IC$_{50}$ values of 1.00, 0.63, 0.73 and 0.58 for the cell lines MCF-7, A549, K562, and HL-60 respectively.

3.12. Antimicrobial Assay

The antimicrobial activities against pathogenic bacteria, *Escherichia coli* ATCC 11775, *Staphylococcus aureus* ATCC 6538, *Pseudomonas aeruginosa* ATCC10145, *Clostridium perfringens* CGMCC 1.0876 and *Bacillus subtilis* CGMCC 1.3376, as well as the pathogenic fungus, *Candida albicans* ATCC 10231 were evaluated by an agar dilution method [21]. The tested strains were cultivated in LB agar plates for bacteria and YPD agar plates for *C. albicans* at 37 °C. Compounds **1**, **3** and **4** and positive controls were dissolved in MeOH at different concentrations from 100 to 0.05 μg/mL by the continuous 2-fold dilution methods. A 10 μL quantity of test solution was absorbed by a paper disk (5 mm diameter) and placed on the assay plates. After 12 h incubation, zones of inhibition (mm in diameter) were recorded. The minimum inhibitory concentrations (MICs) were defined as the lowest concentration at which no microbial growth could be observed. Ciprofloxacin lactate (for bacteria) and ketoconazole (for fungus) were used as positive control for *E. coli*, *S. aureus*, *P. aeruginosa*, *C. perfringens*, *B. subtilis*, *C. albicans* with MIC values of 1.9, 1.9, 3.8, 1.9, 0.94, and 0.02 µM, respectively.

4. Conclusions

In summary, we identified four polyene macrolactams (**1–4**) from a deep-sea sediment-derived *Streptomyces* strain, OUCMDZ-3159. Compounds **1** and **2** with 20-membered or larger ring moieties existed a keto-enol tautomerism in the DMSO solution or pyridine solution. The abiotic formation of **2** and **4** from **1** was clarified through a package of heat and light induced intramolecular pericyclic reactions. This study indicated that light was a key factor that made the polyene macrolactams unstable at rt. The results provide ideas for the research on the non-enzymatic formation of polycyclic macrolactams.

Supplementary Materials: The following are available online at https://www.mdpi.com/1660-3397/19/1/13/s1. Tables S1–S3: NMR data for compounds **4**, **1a**, **1b**, **1c** and **2a** and X-ray crystallographic analysis. Figure S1–S48: NMR and HRESIMS spectra.

Author Contributions: P.W. performed the experiments for the isolation, structure elucidation, reactions under different conditions, and biological activity assay and prepared the draft manuscript; D.W. jointly contributed to isolation, preparation of compounds and performed HRESIMS and ECD experiments. R.Z. performed the fermentation of the strain; Y.W. and F.K. participated in the structure elucidation; P.F. and W.Z. supervised the research work and revised the manuscript. All authors have read and agreed to the published version of the manuscript.

Funding: This research received no external funding.

Institutional Review Board Statement: Not applicable.

Informed Consent Statement: Not applicable.

Acknowledgments: This work was financially supported by the National Natural Science Foundation of China (Nos. U1906213, 41876172, 41806086), the National Key R&D Program of China (No. 2018YFC1406705) and the Fundamental Research Funds for the Central Universities (No. 201841006).

Conflicts of Interest: The authors declare no conflict of interest.

References

1. Skellam, E.J.; Stewart, A.K.; Strangman, W.K.; Wright, J.L.C. Identification of micromonolactam, a new polyene macrocyclic lactam from two marine *Micromonospora* strains using chemical and molecular methods: Clarification of the biosynthetic pathway from a glutamate starter unit. *J. Antibiot.* **2013**, *66*, 431–441.
2. Sugiyama, R.; Nishimura, S.; Matsumori, N.; Tsunematsu, Y.; Hattori, A.; Kakeya, H. Structure and biological activity of 8-deoxyheronamide C from a marine-derived *Streptomyces* sp.: Heronamides target saturated hydrocarbon chains in lipid membranes. *J. Am. Chem. Soc.* **2014**, *136*, 5209–5212. [PubMed]
3. Schulze, C.J.; Donia, M.S.; Siqueira-Neto, J.L.; Ray, D.; Raskatov, J.A.; Green, R.E.; McKerrow, J.H.; Fischbach, M.A.; Linington, R.G. Genome-directed lead discovery: Biosynthesis, structure elucidation, and biological evaluation of two families of polyene macrolactams against *Trypanosoma brucei*. *ACS Chem. Biol.* **2015**, *10*, 2373–2381. [PubMed]
4. Genilloud, O. Actinomycetes: Still a source of novel antibiotics. *Nat. Prod. Rep.* **2017**, *34*, 1203–1232.
5. Hoshino, S.; Okada, M.; Awakawa, T.; Asamizu, S.; Onaka, H.; Abe, I. Mycolic acid containing bacterium stimulates tandem cyclization of polyene macrolactam in a lake sediment derived rare actinomycete. *Org. Lett.* **2017**, *19*, 4992–4995.
6. Shin, Y.H.; Beom, J.Y.; Chung, B.; Shin, Y.; Byun, W.S.; Moon, K.; Bae, M.; Lee, S.K.; Oh, K.B.; Shin, J.; et al. Bombyxamycins A and B, cytotoxic macrocyclic lactams from an intestinal bacterium of the silkworm *Bombyx mori*. *Org. Lett.* **2019**, *21*, 1804–1808.
7. Beemelmanns, C.; Ramadhar, T.R.; Kim, K.H.; Klassen, J.L.; Cao, S.; Wyche, T.P.; Hou, Y.; Poulsen, M.; Bugni, T.S.; Currie, C.R.; et al. Macrotermycins A–D, glycosylated macrolactams from a termite-associated *Amycolatopsis* sp. M39. *Org. Lett.* **2017**, *19*, 1000–1003.
8. Nogawa, T.; Okano, A.; Takahashi, S.; Uramoto, M.; Konno, H.; Saito, T.; Osada, H. Verticilactam, a new macrolactam isolated from a microbial metabolite fraction library. *Org. Lett.* **2010**, *12*, 4564–4567.
9. Oh, D.C.; Poulsen, M.; Currie, C.R.; Clardy, J. Sceliphrolactam, a polyene macrocyclic lactam from a wasp-associated *Streptomyces* sp. *Org. Lett.* **2011**, *13*, 752–755.
10. Park, S.H.; Moon, K.; Bang, H.S.; Kim, S.H.; Kim, D.G.; Oh, K.B.; Shin, J.; Oh, D.C. Tripartilactam, a cyclobutane-bearing tricyclic lactam from a *Streptomyces* sp. in a dung beetle's brood ball. *Org. Lett.* **2012**, *14*, 1258–1261.

11. Hoshino, S.; Okada, M.; Wakimoto, T.; Zhang, H.P.; Hayashi, F.; Onaka, H.; Abe, I. Niizalactams A–C, multicyclic macrolactams isolated from combined culture of *Streptomyces* with mycolic acid-containing bacterium. *J. Nat. Prod.* **2015**, *78*, 3011–3017. [CrossRef] [PubMed]
12. Hwang, S.; Kim, E.; Lee, J.; Shin, J.; Yoon, Y.J.; Oh, D.C. Structure revision and the biosynthetic pathway of tripartilactam. *J. Nat. Prod.* **2020**, *83*, 578–583. [CrossRef] [PubMed]
13. Fu, P.; Liu, P.; Li, X.; Wang, Y.; Wang, S.; Hong, K.; Zhu, W. Cyclic bipyridine glycosides from the marine-derived actinomycete *Actinoalloteichus cyanogriseus* WH1-2216-6. *Org. Lett.* **2011**, *13*, 5948–5951. [CrossRef] [PubMed]
14. Fu, P.; Zhu, Y.; Mei, X.; Wang, Y.; Jia, H.; Zhang, C.; Zhu, W. Acyclic congeners from *Actinoalloteichus cyanogriseus* provide insights into cyclic bipyridine glycoside formation. *Org. Lett.* **2014**, *16*, 4264–4267. [CrossRef]
15. Shen, J.; Fan, Y.; Zhu, G.; Chen, H.; Zhu, W.; Fu, P. Polycyclic macrolactams generated via intramolecular diels–alder reactions from an Antarctic *Streptomyces* species. *Org. Lett.* **2019**, *21*, 4816–4820. [CrossRef] [PubMed]
16. Shen, J.; Wang, J.; Chen, H.; Wang, Y.; Zhu, W.; Fu, P. Cyclamenols E and F, two diastereoisomeric bicyclic macrolactams with a cyclopentane moiety from an Antarctic *Streptomyces* species. *Org. Chem. Front.* **2020**, *7*, 310–317. [CrossRef]
17. Seco, J.M.; Quiñoá, E.; Riguera, R. A practical guide for the assignment of the absolute configuration of alcohols, amines and carboxylic acids by NMR. *Tetrahedron Asymmetry* **2001**, *12*, 2915–2925. [CrossRef]
18. Matsumori, N.; Kaneno, D.; Murata, M.; Nakamura, H.; Tachibana, K. Stereochemical determination of acyclic structures based on carbon-proton spin-coupling constants. A method of configuration analysis for natural products. *J. Org. Chem.* **1999**, *64*, 866–876. [CrossRef]
19. Mosmann, T. Rapid colorimetric assay for cellular growth and survival: Application to proliferation and cytotoxicity assays. *J. Immunol. Methods* **1983**, *65*, 55–63. [CrossRef]
20. Xiong, T.; Chen, X.; Wei, H.; Xiao, H. Influence of PJ34 on the genotoxicity induced by melphalan in human multiple myeloma cells. *Arch. Med. Sci.* **2015**, *11*, 301–306. [CrossRef]
21. Zaika, L.L.J. Spices and herbs: Their antimicrobial activity and its determination. *J. Food Safety* **1988**, *9*, 97–118. [CrossRef]

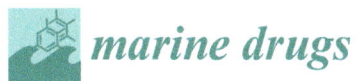

Article

Isolation and Characterization of New Anti-Inflammatory and Antioxidant Components from Deep Marine-Derived Fungus *Myrothecium* sp. Bzo-l062

Xiaojie Lu [1,2,†], Junjie He [1,†], Yanhua Wu [3], Na Du [1], Xiaofan Li [1], Jianhua Ju [4], Zhangli Hu [1,2], Kazuo Umezawa [3,*] and Liyan Wang [1,*]

1 Shenzhen Key Laboratory of Marine Bioresource and Eco-environmental Science, College of Life Sciences and Oceanography, Shenzhen University, Shenzhen 518060, China; luxiaojie@szu.edu.cn (X.L.); hejunjie2017@email.szu.edu.cn (J.H.); duna2017@email.szu.edu.cn (N.D.); lixiaof@szu.edu.cn (X.L.); huzl@szu.edu.cn (Z.H.)
2 Key Laboratory of Optoelectronic Devices and Systems of Ministry of Education and Guangdong Province, College of Optoelectronic Engineering, Shenzhen University, Shenzhen 518060, China
3 Department of Molecular Target Medicine, Aichi Medical University School of Medicine, Nagakute 480-1195, Japan; wu.yanhua.196@mail.aichi-med-u.ac.jp
4 CAS Key Laboratory of Tropical Marine Bio-resources and Ecology, South China Sea Institute of Oceanology, Chinese Academy of Sciences, Guangzhou 510301, China; jju@scsio.ac.cn
* Correspondence: umezawa@aichi-med-u.ac.jp (K.U.); lwang@szu.edu.cn (L.W.); Tel.: +81-561-61-1959 (K.U.); +86-755-2601-2653 (L.W.)
† These authors contributed equally to this work.

Received: 3 November 2020; Accepted: 24 November 2020; Published: 26 November 2020

Abstract: In the present study, four new compounds including a pair of 2-benzoyl tetrahydrofuran enantiomers, namely, (−)-1S-myrothecol (**1a**) and (+)-1R-myrothecol (**1b**), a methoxy-myrothecol racemate (**2**), and an azaphilone derivative, myrothin (**3**), were isolated along with four known compounds (**4**–**7**) from cultures of the deep-sea fungus *Myrothecium* sp. BZO-L062. Enantiomeric compounds **1a** and **1b** were separated through normal-phase chiral high-performance liquid chromatography. The absolute configurations of **1a**, **1b**, and **3** were assigned by ECD spectra. Among them, the new compound **1a** and its enantiomer **1b** exhibited anti-inflammatory activity, inhibited nitric oxide formation in lipopolysaccharide-treated RAW264.7 cells, and exhibited antioxidant activity in the 2,2-azino-bis(3-ethylbenzothiazoline-6-sulfonic acid) and oxygen radical absorbance capacity assays.

Keywords: deep sea marine-derived fungus; *Myrothecium* sp.; myrothecol; nitric oxide (NO); antioxidant activity

1. Introduction

Natural products are a rich source of new drugs and they are frequently used for the discovery and development of new drugs [1]. Natural marine products with unique architectures and distinct biological activities are treasure troves for natural product chemists [2,3]. Among marine organisms, fungi produce a diverse range of biologically active metabolites [3], including polyketides [4–6], terpenoids [7–9], polypeptides [10], and alkaloids [11–13].

Microorganisms of the deep-sea are an attractive source of candidate drugs. While screening inhibitors of lipopolysaccharide (LPS)-induced nitric oxide (NO) production, we recently isolated cyclopenol and cyclopenin from the extract of the fungal strain *Aspergillus* sp. SCSIOW2 collected from a depth of approximately 2000 m in the sea [14]. At non-toxic concentrations, these compounds inhibited LPS-induced NO production and IL-6 secretion in RAW264.7 cells. This inhibitory effect of cyclopenol and cyclopenin was attributed to the suppression of the upstream signal of NF-B activation. These compounds also suppressed the expression of IL-1β, IL-6, and iNOS in microglia cells (macrophages in the mouse brain) [14]. In Alzheimer's disease, amyloid β-peptide induces inflammation in the brain. Between the two compounds, cyclopenin showed ameliorative effects in an in vivo Alzheimer's model using flies [14].

To explore new bioactive secondary metabolites from deep marine-derived fungi [15–17], a fungal strain, *Myrothecium* sp. BZO-L062, isolated from sediment samples collected from the sea bottom near Yongxing Island, was used for chemical investigation. Seven pure components, including four new compounds (**1a**, **1b**, **2**, and **3**), were isolated and identified from the ethyl acetate extract of the fungus (Figure 1). The absolute configurations of the new compounds (**1a**, **1b**, and **3**) were assigned by comparison of their experimental CD spectra with the theoretically calculated spectra. The NO production inhibitory activity and antioxidant activity of the new compounds were also evaluated. Known compounds **4–7** were identified as terreinol (**4**) [18], 3,5-dihydroxy-4-methylbenzoic acid methyl ester (**5**), 5-hydroxymethyl-2-furoic acid (**6**) [19], and 5-hydroxymethyl-2-furancarboxylic acid methyl ester (**7**) [20] by comparing their spectroscopic data with those previously reported.

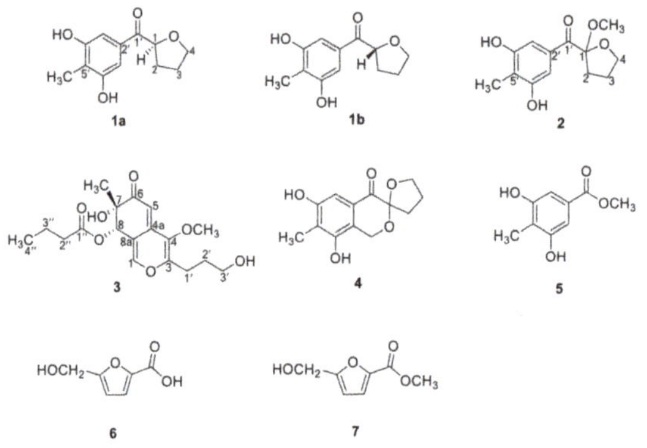

Figure 1. Compounds **1–7** isolated from *Myrothecium* sp. BZO-L062, including (−)-(1*S*)-myrotheciol (**1a**), (+)-(1*R*)-myrotheciol (**1b**), 1-methoxy-myrotheciol (**2**), myrothin (**3**), terreinol (**4**), 3,5-dihydroxy-4-methylbenzoic acid methyl ester (**5**), 5-hydroxymethyl-2-furoic acid (**6**), and 5-hydroxymethyl-2-furancarboxylic acid methyl ester (**7**).

2. Results and Discussion

The molecular formula of **1** was determined as $C_{12}H_{14}O_4$ by high-resolution electrospray ionization mass spectrometry (HRESIMS) at m/z 223.0958 [M + H]$^+$ and 245.0780 [M + Na]$^+$ (calculated for $C_{12}H_{15}O_4{}^+$, 223.0965; $C_{12}H_{14}O_4Na^+$, 245.0784) (Figure S1). ^{1}H NMR, ^{13}C NMR, and 2D-NMR data of **1** (Table 1, Figures S2–S8) revealed the presence of 12 resonance signals, including those for one sp^3 methyl, one sp^3 oxygenated methine, three sp^3 methylenes, two symmetric sp^2 methines, two symmetric sp^2 oxygenated quaternary carbons, two sp^2 quaternary carbons, and one ketone carbonyl carbon. The ^{1}H-^{1}H correlation spectroscopy (COSY) data from H-1 to H$_2$-4 and the ^{1}H-^{13}C heteronuclear multiple bond correlations (HMBC) from H-1 to oxygenated C-4 and from H$_2$-4 to C-1 suggested the presence of a tetrahydro-2-furanyl moiety (Table 1 and Figure 2). The four aromatic carbon signals indicated the presence of one symmetrically substituted benzene ring. The HMBC experiment correlations confirmed the presence of a 3,5-dihydroxy-4-methyl benzoyl moiety (Table 1 and Figure 2). Finally, the key HMBC correlations from H$_2$-2 to C-1 and from H-1 to C-2 allowed the linkage of the 3,5-dihydroxy-4-methyl benzoyl and tetrahydro-2-furanyl groups (Table 1 and Figure 2). Accordingly, **1** was established as (3,5-dihydroxy-4-methylphenyl)-(tetrahydro-2-furanyl)methanone and denoted as a myrotheciol.

Table 1. ^{1}H NMR (600 MHz) and ^{13}C NMR (150 MHz) spectral data of 1.

No.	δ_C	δ_H, Mult. (J in Hz)	^{1}H-^{1}H COSY	HMBC
1	79.1	5.09, dd (8.4, 5.6)	2	C-2,3,4
2	29.0	2.17, m; 1.92, m	1,3	C-1,3,4,1'
3	25.2	1.84, m	2,4	C-1,2,4
4	68.4	3.81, t (6.7)	3	C-1,2,3
1'	198.0	-		
2'	132.7	-		
3',7'	106.1	6.92, s		C-1',2',4'(6'),5'
4',6'	156.1	-		
5'	116.7	-		
4'–OH/6'–OH	-	9.51, s		C-3',4',5'/C-5',6',7'
5'–CH$_3$	8.9	1.99, s		C-4',5',6'

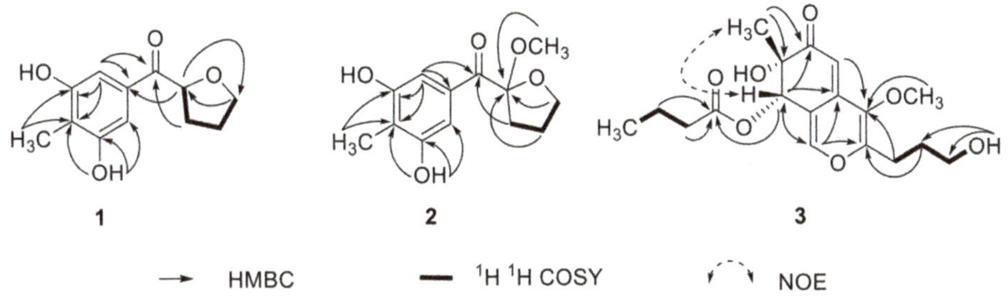

Figure 2. Key 2D NMR correlations of 1–3.

The absence of the Cotton effect in the CD spectrum and zero specific rotation indicated that 1 was a racemate. Generally, enantiomers are more advantageous than racemates for drug development. To detect the enantiomers of 1, chiral HPLC was performed using a Chiralpak IC column; the HPLC results showed two separate peaks (Figure S9). The two enantiomers, (−)-1a and (+)-1b, were obtained in a ratio of 1:1. (−)-1a and (+)-1b showed mirror image-like CD curves (Figure 3) and opposite specific rotations (1a: $[\alpha]_D^{20}$ − 25.3; 1b: $[\alpha]_D^{20}$ + 26.3). The experimental CD spectra of 1a were consistent with the theoretically calculated ECD spectrum of the 1-S enantiomer with four Cotton effects observed at 237 nm (positive), 270 nm (positive), 310 nm (negative), and 348 nm (positive) (Figure 3). In contrast, the CD spectrum of 1b was consistent with the ECD spectrum of the 1-R enantiomer but different from that of 1-S with three negative Cotton effects at 237 nm, 270 nm, and 348 nm, and one positive Cotton effect at 310 nm. Thus, the absolute configurations of 1a and 1b were assigned as (−)-(1S)-myrotheciol and (+)-(1R)-myrotheciol, respectively (Figure 1).

The molecular formula of 2 was determined as $C_{13}H_{16}O_5$ through HRESIMS at m/z 275.0896 [M + Na]$^+$ (calculated for $C_{13}H_{16}O_5Na^+$, 275.0890), which was 30 mass units larger than 1 (Figure S10). The ^{1}H and ^{13}C NMR data of 2 (Table 2, Figures S11–S16) closely resembled those of 1, except for three major differences: the presence of an additional methoxy group (δ_H 3.09, δ_C 50.2), the absence of a methine proton (δ_H 5.09), and the chemical shift of C-1 (from δ_C 79.1 to 109.5); these differences indicated the substitution of the methine proton at C-1 by a methoxy group. The position of the new methoxy group was confirmed by HMBC correlation from 1-OMe to C-1 (Table 2 and Figure 2). Thus, 2 was established as 1-methoxy-myrotheciol. The structure of 2 was validated through a detailed analysis of 2D NMR data (Table 2 and Figure 2).

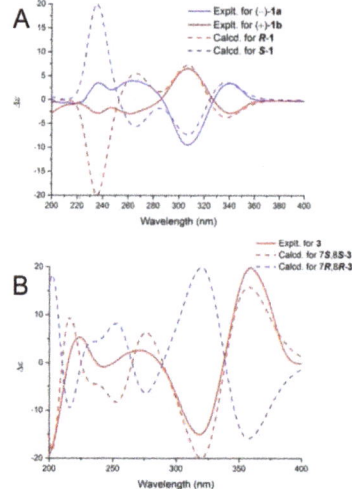

Figure 3. ECD spectra of compounds **1a** and **1b** (**A**), and **3**(**B**).

Table 2. ^{1}H NMR (600 MHz) and ^{13}C NMR (150 MHz) spectral data of **2**.

No.	δ_C	δ_H, Mult. (J in Hz)	^{1}H-^{1}H COSY	HMBC
1	109.5	-		
2	34.6	2.13, m	3	C-1,3,4,1'
3	24.0	1.88, m; 2.01, m	2,4	C-1,2,4
4	68.1	3.96, m	3	C-1,2,3
1'	194.8	-		
2'	131.7	-		
3',7'	107.3	7.09, s		C-1',2',4'(6'),5'
4',6'	155.9	-		
5'	116.7	-		
1-OCH$_3$	50.2	3.09, s		C-1
4'-OH/6'-OH	-	9.47, s		C-3',4',5'/C-5',6',7'
5'-CH$_3$	8.9	1.98, s		C-4',5',6'

Compound **2** was also considered as a racemic mixture based on the zero specific rotation and absence of the Cotton effect in its CD spectrum. The chiral HPLC performed using the same condition as that used for **1** revealed two peaks, attributable to **2a** and **2b**, at a ratio of approximately 1:1 (Figure S17). However, due to the limited sample size, further isolation was not carried out.

(+)-HRESIMS at m/z 353.1599 [M + H]$^+$ and 375.1418 [M + Na]$^+$ (calculated for C$_{18}$H$_{25}$O$_7{}^+$, 353.1595; C$_{18}$H$_{24}$O$_7$Na$^+$, 375.1414) revealed the molecular formula of **3** as C$_{18}$H$_{24}$O$_7$ (Figure S18). The 1D- and 2DNMR results revealed the presence of one sp^3 oxygenated quaternary carbon, one sp^3 oxygenated methine, two sp^2 aromatic methines, four sp^2 quaternary carbons, one ketone carbonyl carbon, one methoxy group, and one angular methyl group (Table 3 and Figures S19–25). Other than these signals, the ^{1}H-^{1}H COSY correlations from H-2" to H-4", along with the HMBC correlations from H-2" and 3" to C-1" (Table 3 and Figure 2) indicated the presence of the butyl ester fragment. The ^{1}H-^{1}H COSY correlations from H-1 to 3-OH corresponded to the hydroxypropyl fragment (Table 3, Figure 2). The NMR data of the core structure of **3** closely resembled those of C-8 dihydro-azaphilone [21,22]. Careful HMBC analysis confirmed this structure (Table 3 and Figure 2). Finally, the key HMBC correlation from H-8 to C-1"connected the butyl ester side chain to C-8, that from H-1 and H-2 to

C-3 connected the hydroxypropyl group moiety to C-3, and that from 4-OCH$_3$ to C-4 connected the methoxy group to C-4 (Table 3 and Figure 2). Accordingly, 3 was established as myrothin (Figure 1).

Table 3. ^{1}H NMR (600 MHz) and ^{13}C NMR (150 MHz) data of 3.

No.	δ$_C$	δ$_H$, Mult. (J in Hz)	^{1}H-^{1}H COSY	HMBC
1	146.9	7.66, d (1.2)		C-3,4a,8,8a
3	154.7	-		
4	138.3	-		
4a	139.6	-		
5	99.7	5.28, d (1.2)		C-4,7,8a
6	196.5	-		
7	73.29	-		
8	73.30	5.54, s		C-1,4a,6,7,8a,1″
8a	116.5	-		
1′	24.2	2.58, m	2′	C-3,4,2′,3′
2′	29.6	1.68, m	1′,3′	C-3,1′,3′
3′	59.88	3.44, m	2′,3′-OH	C-1′,2′
3′-OH	-	4.58, t (5.1)	3′	C-2′,3′
4-OCH$_3$	59.94	3.62, s		C-4
7-CH$_3$	23.4	1.16, s		C-6,7
7-OH	-	5.07, s		C-6,7,7-CH$_3$
1″	172.2	-		
2″	35.4	2.26, t (7.2)	3″	C-1″,3″,4″
3″	17.9	1.49, m	2″, 4″	C-1″,2″,4″
4″	13.2	0.82, t (7.4)	3″	C-2″,3″

The relative configuration of 3 at C-7 and C-8 was assigned by nuclear overhauser effect spectroscopy (NOESY) correlations. The strong NOESY correlation between 7-CH$_3$ and H-8 indicated that 7-CH$_3$ and H-8 occupied the same side of the ring (Figure 2 and Figure S25). Thus, the stereo-configurations of C-7 and C-8 are either S,S or R,R. The experimental ECD curve of 3 was consistent with that of the 7S, 8S epimer (Figure 3). The chiral carbons C-7 and C-8 were thus determined as 7S and 8S.

LPS-induced NO production in RAW264.7 cells was used to evaluate the anti-inflammatory activity of different compounds [14]. NO is produced by NF-κB-dependent inducible NO synthase. All the isolated compounds were evaluated for cytotoxicity and for their effects on LPS-induced NO production. Among all the tested compounds, only two new compounds (1a and 1b) significantly inhibited LPS-induced NO production at non-toxic concentrations (Figure 4).

Antioxidant activities were measured through 2,2-azino-bis(3-ethylbenzothiazoline-6-sulfonic acid) (ABTS) scavenging activity, 1,1-diphenyl-2-picrylhydrazyl (DPPH) scavenging capacity, and the oxygen radical absorbance capacity (ORAC) assay. As shown in Table 4, new compounds 1a and 1b exhibited antioxidant activity in the ABTS assay with EC$_{50}$ of 1.20 and 1.41 µgmL^{-1}, respectively, which were comparable with EC$_{50}$ values of the positive controls L-ascorbic acid (1.55 µgmL^{-1}) and trolox (1.61 µgmL^{-1}). In the ORAC assay, the antioxidant ability was expressed as µmol trolox equivalents per µmol of sample solution. Compounds 1a and 1b showed high antioxidant activity (1.41 µM trolox/µM for 1a and 1.19 µM trolox/µM for 1b). Generally, the scavenging activities of ABTS are significantly higher than the scavenging activities of DPPH in phenolic compounds [23]. Compounds 1a and 1b did not show antioxidant activity in the DPPH assay, even at the highest concentration of 10 µgmL^{-1}.

In the present research, we isolated several compounds including new structures from a deep-sea fungus. We found cellular anti-inflammatory activity in 1a and 1b. Microorganisms often produce useful compounds for therapy. However, the role of these compounds on producing organisms is not clear. At the beginning of antibiotic research, antibiotics are considered to protect the producing organisms by killing their enemy microorganisms. But later, many enzyme inhibitors such as pepstatin and leupeptin were discovered from the secondary metabolites of *Streptomyces*, and they showed no antibiotic activity. Therefore, it is unlikely that these secondary metabolites are useful for the producers. From this point of view, new compounds, **1a** and **1b**, may be remnants of microorganisms in their evolution.

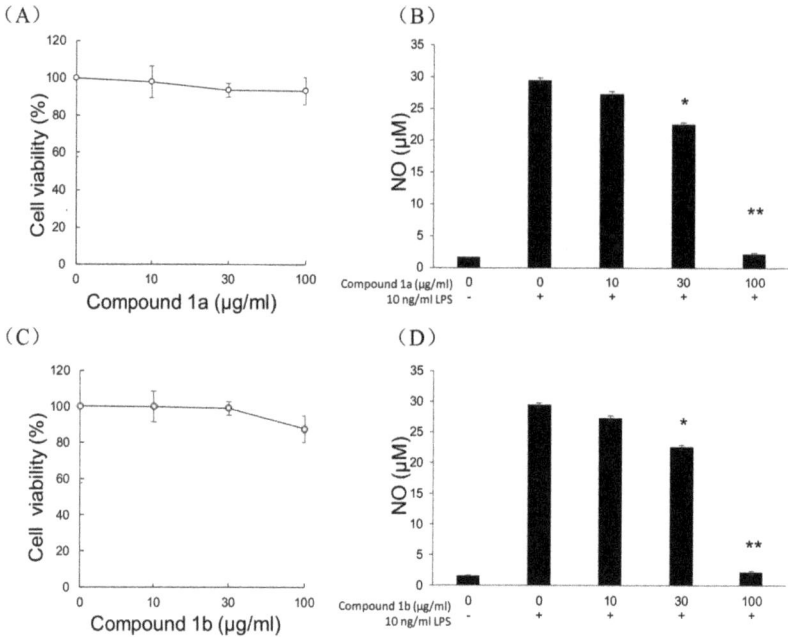

Figure 4. NO production inhibitory activity of **1a** and **1b** in RAW264.7 cells. Effect of **1a** (**A**) or **1b** (**C**) on the viability of RAW264.7 cells. Inhibition of LPS-induced NO production by **1a** (**B**) or **1b** (**D**). Values represent the means ± SEM of three independent experiments. *, $p < 0.05$; **, $p < 0.001$ vs. control.

Table 4. Antioxidant activities of **1a** and **1b**.

Compounds	ABTS	ORAC
	EC_{50}, µg/mL	µM Trolox Equivalent/µM
1a	1.20 ± 0.18	1.41 ± 0.27
1b	1.41 ± 0.19	1.19 ± 0.19
L-Ascorbic acid	1.55 ± 0.15	0.35 ± 0.14
Trolox	1.61 ± 0.09	NA

3. Materials and Methods

3.1. General Experimental Procedures

Optical rotations were recorded on an Anton Paar MCP-100 polarimeter (Anton Paar GmbH, Graz, Austria). ECD spectra were measured on a JASCO-810 spectropolarimeter (JASCO Corporation, Tokyo, Japan). UV spectra were obtained on a UV-1800 spectrophotometer (Shimadzu Corporation, Tokyo, Japan). IR spectra were recorded on a Nicolet Avatar 330 FT-IR spectrometer (Thermo Scientific, Waltham, MA, USA) using KBr disks. NMR spectra were acquired on a Bruker ASCEND 500 MHz or 600 MHz NMR magnet system (Bruker, Ettlingen, Germany) using tetramethylsilane (TMS) as the internal standard. HRESIMS was performed using a Triple TOF 6600 (AB SCIEX LLC, Framingham, MA, USA). Column chromatography (CC) was conducted using silica gel (200–300 mesh,

Qingdao Marine Chemical Factory, Qingdao, China) and Sephadex LH-20 (Amersham Pharmacia Biotech, Piscataway, NJ, USA). Thin-layer chromatography (TLC) was performed on Merck TLC plates silica gel 60 F_{254} and silica gel 60 RP-18 F_{254S} (Merck Millipore Corporation, Darmstadt, Germany). HPLC was carried out on a Shimadzu LC-16P HPLC system (Shimadzu Corporation, Tokyo, Japan) using YMC-pack Pro C18 Column (4.6 × 250 mm, 5 μm; 10 × 250 mm, 5 μm; YMC Co., Ltd., Kyoto, Japan) for analysis and semi-preparation. Optical pure compounds were prepared using a DAICEL Chiralpak IC column (250 mm × 4.6 mm, 5 μm; YMC Co., Ltd., Kyoto, Japan). All the chemical reagents for isolation were either of analytical (Damao Chemical Factory, Tianjin, China) or HPLC grade (Kermel Chemical Co., Ltd., Tianjin, China).

3.2. Fungal Material

The fungus *Myrothecium* sp. BZO-L062 used in this study was isolated from a deep-sea (2130 m depth) sediment sample collected from an area close to Yongxing Island, China. The strain was identified as *Myrothecium* sp. based on the morphological features and internal transcribed spacer sequence analysis. This strain was deposited at the Marine Natural Products Laboratory, College of Life Sciences and Oceanography, Shenzhen University, Shenzhen, China.

3.3. Fermentation and Extraction

The fungus *Myrothecium* sp. BZO-L062 was activated on petri dishes containing potato dextrose agar supplemented with 3% sea salt at 28 °C for three days [24]. Agar plugs were inoculated in a 500 mL Erlenmeyer flask containing 150 mL of liquid potato dextrose culture medium [24] supplemented with 3% sea salt as seed cultures and were incubated at 28 °C on a rotary shaker at 180 rpm for three days. Large-scale fermentation (70 L) was conducted using the same medium as that for seed cultures at 28 °C and 180 rpm for seven days. After seven days, the fermentation broth was filtered through cheesecloth to separate the supernatant from the mycelia. The supernatant was then concentrated to 8 L and successively extracted three times with EtOAc (3 × 8 L), yielding a crude extract (40.0 g).

3.4. Isolation and Purification

The crude extract was separated using silica gel CC through CH_2Cl_2/MeOH gradient elution (100:0, 100:1, 100:5, 100:10, 100:20, 100:50, and 0:100; 600 mL each) and was grouped into nine fractions (Fr.) based on the TLC analysis (Fr.1 to Fr.9). Fr.3 was purified by semi-preparative HPLC (28% MeCN/H_2O, flow rate 3 mLmin^{-1}) to yield **4** (t_R 16.2 min, 10.1 mg). Fr.4 was subjected to HPLC using a medium-pressure octadecyl-silica (ODS) column and separated with MeOH/H_2O (20–100%) into five fractions (Fr.4.1–Fr.4.5). Fr.4.1 was further fractionated by HPLC (5% MeOH/H_2O, a flow rate of 3 mLmin^{-1}) to obtain **6** (t_R 15.0 min, 5.0 mg) and **7** (t_R 24.0 min, 5.0 mg). Fr.4.2 was purified by HPLC (25% MeOH/H_2O, a flow rate of 3 mLmin^{-1}) to obtain **3** (t_R 21.0 min, 1.0 mg). Fr.4.3 was refined by HPLC (25% MeCN/H_2O, a flow rate of 3 mLmin^{-1}) to obtain **2** (t_R 20.0 min, 1.4 mg). Finally, Fr.5 was subjected to HPLC (17% MeCN/H_2O, flow rate 3 mLmin^{-1}) to obtain **1** (t_R 20.0 min, 14.2 mg) and **5** (t_R 21.2 min, 10.2 mg).

The racemic compound **1** was resolved into enantiomers (−)-**1a** (3.0 mg, t_R 10.2 min) and (+)-**1b** (3.6 mg, t_R 18.1 min) using a chiral HPLC equipped with a DAICEL® Cellulose Chiralpak IC column (5 μm, 4.6 × 250 mm) using *n*-hexane-ethanol (89:11) as mobile phase at a flow rate of 1 mLmin^{-1}.

3.5. Spectral Data of the Compounds

3.5.1. (±)-Myrothecol (**1**)

Myrothecol (**1**) is a colorless oil; $[\alpha]_D^{20}$ 0° (*c* 0.1, MeOH); UV (MeOH) λ_{max} (log ε) 280 nm (7.18) and 218 nm (7.46); IR (KBr) ν_{max} 3325, 2956, 1678, 1591, 1423, 1325, 1198, 1088, 1040, 934, and 851; HRESIMS *m/z* 223.0958 [M+H]$^+$, 245.0780 [M+Na]$^+$ (calculated for $C_{12}H_{15}O_4$, 223.0965; $C_{12}H_{14}O_4Na$, 245.0784); for ^1H NMR (DMSO-d_6, 600 MHz) and ^{13}C NMR (DMSO-d_6, 150 MHz) spectral data, see Table 1.

(−)-**1a**: $[\alpha]_D^{20}$ −25.3° (c 0.3, MeOH); ECD (2.3 mM, MeOH) λ_{max} ($\Delta\varepsilon$) 237 nm (+0.49), 262 nm (+0.54), 307 nm (−1.27), 341 nm (+0.48). (+)-**1b**: $[\alpha]_D^{20}$ + 26.3° (c 0.27, MeOH); ECD (2.3 mM, MeOH) λ_{max} ($\Delta\varepsilon$) 237 nm (−0.38), 262 nm (−0.39), 307 nm (+0.88), and 341 nm (−0.37).

3.5.2. Methoxy-myrothecol (2)

Methoxy-myrothecol (**2**) is a colorless oil; $[\alpha]_D^{20}$ 0° (c 0.1, MeCN); UV (MeOH) λ_{max}(log ε) 285 nm (6.99) and 218 nm (7.24); HRESIMS m/z 275.0896 [M+Na]$^+$ (calculated for $C_{13}H_{16}O_5Na$, 275.0890); HRESIMS m/z 353.1599 [M+H]$^+$, 375.1418 [M+Na]$^+$ (calculated for $C_{18}H_{25}O_7$, 353.1595; $C_{18}H_{24}O_7Na$, 375.1414); for ^{1}H NMR (DMSO-d_6, 600 MHz) and ^{13}C NMR (DMSO-d_6, 150 MHz) spectral data, see Table 2.

3.5.3. Myrothin (3)

Myrothin (**3**) is a light-yellow colored oil; UV (MeOH) λ_{max} (log ε) 246 nm (3.13) and 350 nm (3.56); IR (KBr) ν_{max} 3405, 2925, 2376, 2316, 1621, 1385, 1036, 910, 790, 731, and 635 cm^{-1}; HRESIMS m/z 353.1599 [M+H]$^+$, 375.1418 [M+Na]$^+$, 727.2948 [2M+Na]$^+$ (calculated for $C_{18}H_{25}O_7$, 353.1595; $C_{18}H_{24}O_7Na$, 375.1414; $C_{36}H_{48}O_{14}Na$, 727.2936); for ^{1}H NMR (DMSO-d_6, 600 MHz) and ^{13}C NMR (DMSO-d_6, 150 MHz) spectral data, see Table 3. $[\alpha]_D^{20}$ + 15.7°; ECD (2.8 mM, MeOH) λ_{max} ($\Delta\varepsilon$) 224 nm (+0.7), 243 nm (−0.11), 271 nm (+0.34), 319 nm (+1.96), and 359 nm (+2.59).

3.6. ECD Calculation

The conformational distribution search was conducted with the MMFF94 molecular mechanics force field in Spartan 12 software (Wavefunction Inc., Irvine, CA, USA). The lowest energy conformers within the 5-kcalmol^{-1} energy window were optimized using the Gaussian 09 program [25]. TDDFT calculations for all optimized conformers were performed at the B3LYP/6-31G (d, p) level. The ECD spectra were generated using the software SpecDis [26].

3.7. MTT and NO Production Assay

MTT and NO production inhibitory activities of the isolated compounds in RAW264.7 cells were determined as reported previously [14].

3.8. Antioxidant Activity

The ABTS and DPPH scavenging assays were carried out as reported earlier [23]. L-ascorbic acid and trolox were used as positive controls. The ORAC assay was conducted according to a previously reported protocol [27]. The results were expressed as μmol Trolox equivalents per μmol of sample solution.

4. Conclusions

In this study, four new components, (−)-1S-myrothecol (**1a**), (+)-1R-myrothecol (**1b**), methoxy-myrothecol (**2**), and myrothin (**3**), along with four known compounds (**4–7**), were isolated from the deep-sea fungus *Myrothecium* sp. BZO-L062. The enantiomers **1a** and **1b** were purified by chiral HPLC. The absolute configurations of **1a**, **1b**, and **3** were determined by the calculated ECD.

Among these compounds, new compounds **1a** and **1b** showed anti-inflammatory and antioxidant activities at non-toxic concentrations. Derivatives of these compounds could be potent and safe and may be useful for the development of new anti-inflammatory agents.

Supplementary Materials: The following are available online at http://www.mdpi.com/1660-3397/18/12/597/s1, Figure S1: HR-ESI MS spectrum of compound 1, Figure S2–S8: 1D and 2D NMR spectra of compound 1, Figure S9: Chiral separation of racemic 1, Figure S10: HR-ESI MS spectrum of compound 2, Figure S11–16: 1D and 2D NMR spectra of compound 2, Figure S17: Chiral separation of racemic 2, Figure S18: HR-ESI MS spectrum of compound 3, Figure S19–S25: 1D and 2D NMR spectra of compound 3.

Author Contributions: The contributions of the authors are as follows: X.L. (Xiaojie Lu) was involved in performing fermentation, extraction, structure elucidation, and manuscript preparation; J.H. and N.D. were involved in compound isolation and data acquisition; Y.W. contributed to the evaluation of bioactivities; X.L. (Xiaofan Li), J.J., and Z.H. were involved in manuscript revision; K.U. was involved in the evaluation of biological data and manuscript preparation. L.W. was involved in experimental design, manuscript preparation, supervision, and funding acquisition. All authors have read and agreed to the published version of the manuscript.

Funding: This research was financially supported by the National Key Research and Development Project 2019YFC0312501 and 2018YFA0902504; the Science and Technology Project of Shenzhen City, Shenzhen Bureau of Science, Technology, and Information under Grant JCYJ20180305123659726; and by the Interdisciplinary Innovation Team Project of Shenzhen University. This research was also supported by AMED under Grant No. JP18fk0310118 of Japan.

Acknowledgments: The authors thank the Instrumentation Analysis Center of Shenzhen University for help in acquiring NMR and MS data.

Conflicts of Interest: K.U. and Y.W. belong to the laboratory supported by Shenzhen Wanhe Pharmaceutical Co., Ltd, Shenzhen, China, Meiji Seika Pharma Co., Ltd, Tokyo, Japan, Fukuyu Medical Corporation, Nisshin, Japan, and Brunaise Co., Ltd, Nagoya, Japan. The authors declare no conflict of interest.

References

1. Newman, D.J.; Cragg, G.M. Natural products as sources of new drugs over the nearly four decades from 01/1981 to 09/2019. *J. Nat. Prod.* **2020**, *83*, 770–803. [CrossRef]
2. Blunt, J.W.; Carroll, A.R.; Copp, B.R.; Davis, R.A.; Keyzers, R.A.; Prinsep, M.R. Marine natural products. *Nat. Prod. Rep.* **2018**, *35*, 8–53. [CrossRef]
3. Carroll, A.R.; Copp, B.R.; Davis, R.A.; Keyzers, R.A.; Prinsep, M.R. Marine natural products. *Nat. Prod. Rep.* **2020**, *37*, 175–223. [CrossRef] [PubMed]
4. Zhang, P.P.; Deng, Y.L.; Lin, X.J.; Chen, B.; Li, J.; Liu, H.J.; Chen, S.H.; Liu, L. Anti-inflammatory mono- and dimeric sorbicillinoids from the marine-derived fungus *Trichoderma reesei* 4670. *J. Nat. Prod.* **2019**, *82*, 947–957. [CrossRef] [PubMed]
5. El-Kashef, D.H.; Daletos, G.; Plenker, M.; Hartmann, R.; Proksch, P. Polyketides and a dihydroquinolone alkaloid from a marine-derived strain of the fungus *Metarhizium marquandii*. *J. Nat. Prod.* **2019**, *82*, 2460–2469. [CrossRef]
6. Yang, B.Y.; He, Y.; Lin, S.; Zhang, J.W.; Li, H.Q.; Wang, J.P.; Hu, Z.X.; Zhong, Y.H. Antimicrobial dolabellanes and atranones from a marine-derived strain of the toxigenic fungus *Stachybotrys chartarum*. *J. Nat. Prod.* **2019**, *82*, 1923–1929. [CrossRef] [PubMed]
7. Fang, W.; Wang, J.J.; Wang, J.F.; Shi, L.Q.; Li, K.L.; Lin, X.P.; Min, Y.; Yang, B.; Tang, L.; Liu, Y.H.; et al. Cytotoxic and antibacterial eremophilane sesquiterpenes from the marine-derived fungus *Cochliobolus lunatus* SCSIO41401. *J. Nat. Prod.* **2018**, *81*, 1405–1410. [CrossRef]
8. Wen, H.L.; Yang, X.L.; Liu, Q.; Li, S.J.; Li, Q.; Zang, Y.; Chen, C.M.; Wang, J.W.; Zhu, H.C.; Zhang, Y.H. Structurally diverse meroterpenoids from a marine-derived *Aspergillus* sp. fungus. *J. Nat. Prod.* **2019**, *83*, 99–104. [CrossRef]
9. Zhang, Y.H.; Geng, C.; Zhang, X.W.; Zhu, H.J.; Shao, C.L.; Cao, F.; Wang, C.Y. Discovery of bioactive indole-diketopiperazines from the marine-derived fungus *Penicillium brasilianum* aided by genomic information. *Mar. Drugs* **2019**, *17*, 514. [CrossRef]
10. Luo, X.W.; Lin, Y.; Lu, Y.J.; Zhou, X.F.; Liu, Y.H. Peptides and polyketides isolated from the marine sponge-derived fungus *Aspergillus terreus* SCSIO 41008. *Chin. J. Nat. Med.* **2019**, *17*, 149–154. [CrossRef]
11. Chamni, S.; Sirimangkalakitti, N.; Chanvorachote, P.; Saito, N.; Suwanborirux, K. Chemistry of renieramycins. 17. A new generation of renieramycins: Hydroquinone 5-*O*-monoester analogues of renieramycin M as potential cytotoxic agents against non-small-cell lung cancer cells. *J. Nat. Prod.* **2017**, *80*, 1541–1547. [CrossRef] [PubMed]
12. Li, C.J.; Chen, P.N.; Li, H.J.; Mahmud, T.; Wu, D.L.; Xu, J.; Lan, W.J. Potential antidiabetic fumiquinazoline alkaloids from the marine-derived fungus *Scedosporium apiospermum* F41-1. *J. Nat. Prod.* **2020**, *83*, 1082–1091. [CrossRef] [PubMed]
13. Wang, J.J.; Chen, F.M.; Liu, Y.C.; Liu, Y.X.; Li, K.L.; Yang, X.L.; Liu, S.W.; Zhou, X.F.; Wang, J. Spirostaphylotrichin X from a marine-derived fungus as an anti-influenza agent targeting RNA polymerase PB2. *J. Nat. Prod.* **2018**, *81*, 2722–2730. [CrossRef] [PubMed]

14. Wang, L.; Li, M.; Lin, Y.; Du, S.; Liu, Z.; Ju, J.; Suzuki, H.; Sawada, M.; Umezawa, K. Inhibition of cellular inflammatory mediator production and amelioration of learning deficit in flies by deep sea *Aspergillus*-derived cyclopenin. *J. Antibiot.* **2020**, *73*, 622–629. [CrossRef] [PubMed]
15. Zhou, X.; Fang, P.; Tang, J.; Wu, Z.; Li, X.; Li, S.; Wang, Y.; Liu, G.; He, Z.; Gou, D.; et al. A novel cyclic dipeptide from deep marine-derived fungus *Aspergillus* sp. SCSIOW2. *Nat. Prod. Res.* **2016**, *30*, 52–57. [CrossRef] [PubMed]
16. Li, X.F.; Xia, Z.Y.; Tang, J.Q.; Wu, J.H.; Tong, J.; Li, M.J.; Ju, J.H.; Chen, H.R.; Wang, L.Y. Identification and biological evaluation of secondary metabolites from marine derived fungi-*Aspergillus* sp. SCSIOW3, cultivated in the presence of epigenetic modifying agents. *Molecules* **2017**, *22*, 1302. [CrossRef]
17. Wang, L.Y.; Li, M.J.; Tang, J.Q.; Li, X.F. Eremophilane sesquiterpenes from a deep marine-derived fungus, *Aspergillus* sp. SCSIOW2, cultivated in the presence of epigenetic modifying agents. *Molecules* **2016**, *21*, 473. [CrossRef]
18. Macedo, F.C.; Porto, A.L.M.; Marsaioli, A.J. Terreinol—A novel metabolite from *Aspergillus terreus*: Structure and ^{13}C labeling. *Tetrahedron Lett.* **2004**, *45*, 53–55. [CrossRef]
19. Matsui, T.; Kudo, A.; Tokuda, S.; Matsumoto, K.; Hosoyama, H. Identification of a new natural vasorelaxatant compound, (+)-osbeckic acid, from rutin-free tartary buckwheat extract. *J. Agric. Food. Chem.* **2010**, *58*, 10876–10879. [CrossRef]
20. Schmuck, C.; Machon, U. 2-(Guanidiniocarbonyl)furans as a new class of potential anion hosts: Synthesis and first binding studies. *Eur. J. Org. Chem.* **2006**, *19*, 4385–4392. [CrossRef]
21. Steyn, P.S.; Vleggaar, R. The structure of dihydrodeoxy-8-epi-austdiol and the absolute configuration of the azaphilones. *J. Chem. Soc. Perkin Trans. 1* **1976**, 204–206. [CrossRef]
22. Nukina, M.; Marumo, S. Lunatoic acid A and B, aversion factor and its related metabolite of *Cochliobolus lunata*. *Tetrahedron Lett.* **1977**, *18*, 2603–2606. [CrossRef]
23. Bai, Y.; Chang, J.; Xu, Y.; Cheng, D.; Liu, H.; Zhao, Y.; Yu, Z. Antioxidant and myocardial preservation activities of natural phytochemicals from mung bean (*Vigna radiata* L.) seeds. *J. Agric. Food. Chem.* **2016**, *64*, 4648–4655. [CrossRef] [PubMed]
24. Wang, W.; Lee, J.; Kim, K.-J.; Sung, Y.; Park, K.-H.; Oh, E.; Park, C.; Son, Y.-J.; Kang, H. Austalides, osteoclast differentiation inhibitors from a marine-derived strain of the fungus *Penicillium rudallense*. *J. Nat. Prod.* **2019**, *82*, 3083–3088. [CrossRef] [PubMed]
25. Frisch, M.J.; Trucks, G.W.; Schlegel, H.B.; Scuseria, G.E.; Robb, M.A.; Cheeseman, J.R.; Scalmani, G.; Barone, V.; Petersson, G.A.; Nakatsuji, H.; et al. *Gaussian 09 Revision D. 01*; Gaussian Inc.: Wallingford, CT, USA, 2009.
26. Bruhn, T.; Schaumloeffel, A.; Hemberger, Y.; Bringmann, G. SpecDis: Quantifying the comparison of calculated and experimental electronic circular dichroism spectra. *Chirality* **2013**, *25*, 243–249. [CrossRef] [PubMed]
27. Wakamatsu, J.; Stark, T.D.; Hofmann, T. Antioxidative maillard reaction products generated in processed aged garlic extract. *J. Agric. Food. Chem.* **2019**, *67*, 2190–2200. [CrossRef]

Publisher's Note: MDPI stays neutral with regard to jurisdictional claims in published maps and institutional affiliations.

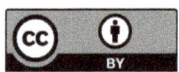

© 2020 by the authors. Licensee MDPI, Basel, Switzerland. This article is an open access article distributed under the terms and conditions of the Creative Commons Attribution (CC BY) license (http://creativecommons.org/licenses/by/4.0/).

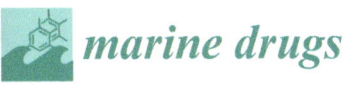

Article

Biotechnological and Ecological Potential of *Micromonospora provocatoris* sp. nov., a Gifted Strain Isolated from the Challenger Deep of the Mariana Trench

Wael M. Abdel-Mageed [1,2], Lamya H. Al-Wahaibi [3], Burhan Lehri [4], Muneera S. M. Al-Saleem [3], Michael Goodfellow [5], Ali B. Kusuma [5,6], Imen Nouioui [5,7], Hariadi Soleh [5], Wasu Pathom-Aree [5], Marcel Jaspars [8] and Andrey V. Karlyshev [4],*

[1] Department of Pharmacognosy, College of Pharmacy, King Saud University, P.O. Box 2457, Riyadh 11451, Saudi Arabia; wabdelmageed@ksu.edu.sa
[2] Department of Pharmacognosy, Faculty of Pharmacy, Assiut University, Assiut 71526, Egypt
[3] Department of Chemistry, Science College, Princess Nourah Bint Abdulrahman University, Riyadh 11671, Saudi Arabia; lhalwahaibi@pnu.edu.sa (L.H.A.-W.); msalsaleem@pnu.edu.sa (M.S.M.A.-S.)
[4] School of Life Sciences Pharmacy and Chemistry, Faculty of Science, Engineering and Computing, Kingston University London, Penrhyn Road, Kingston upon Thames KT1 2EE, UK; b.lehri@hotmail.co.uk
[5] School of Natural and Environmental Sciences, Newcastle University, Newcastle upon Tyne NE1 7RU, UK; Michael.Goodfellow@newcastle.ac.uk (M.G.); ali.budhi.kusuma@uts.ac.id (A.B.K.); ino20@dsmz.de (I.N.); hariadi.soleh@pom.go.id (H.S.); wasu.p@cmu.ac.th (W.P.-T.)
[6] Indonesian Centre for Extremophile Bioresources and Biotechnology (ICEBB), Faculty of Biotechnology, Sumbawa University of Technology, Sumbawa Besar 84371, Indonesia
[7] Leibniz-Institut DSMZ—German Collection of Microorganisms and Cell Cultures, Inhoffenstraße 7B, 38124 Braunschweig, Germany
[8] Marine Biodiscovery Centre, Department of Chemistry, University of Aberdeen, Old Aberdeen AB24 3UE, UK; m.jaspars@abdn.ac.uk
* Correspondence: a.karlyshev@kingston.ac.uk

Citation: Abdel-Mageed, W.M.; Al-Wahaibi, L.H.; Lehri, B.; Al-Saleem, M.S.M.; Goodfellow, M.; Kusuma, A.B.; Nouioui, I.; Soleh, H.; Pathom-Aree, W.; Jaspars, M.; et al. Biotechnological and Ecological Potential of *Micromonospora provocatoris* sp. nov., a Gifted Strain Isolated from the Challenger Deep of the Mariana Trench. *Mar. Drugs* **2021**, *19*, 243. https://doi.org/10.3390/md19050243

Academic Editor: Kazuo Umezawa

Received: 30 March 2021
Accepted: 20 April 2021
Published: 25 April 2021

Publisher's Note: MDPI stays neutral with regard to jurisdictional claims in published maps and institutional affiliations.

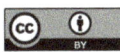

Copyright: © 2021 by the authors. Licensee MDPI, Basel, Switzerland. This article is an open access article distributed under the terms and conditions of the Creative Commons Attribution (CC BY) license (https://creativecommons.org/licenses/by/4.0/).

Abstract: A *Micromonospora* strain, isolate MT25^T, was recovered from a sediment collected from the Challenger Deep of the Mariana Trench using a selective isolation procedure. The isolate produced two major metabolites, *n*-acetylglutaminyl glutamine amide and desferrioxamine B, the chemical structures of which were determined using 1D and 2D-NMR, including ^{1}H-^{15}N HSQC and ^{1}H-^{15}N HMBC 2D-NMR, as well as high resolution MS. A whole genome sequence of the strain showed the presence of ten natural product-biosynthetic gene clusters, including one responsible for the biosynthesis of desferrioxamine B. Whilst 16S rRNA gene sequence analyses showed that the isolate was most closely related to the type strain of *Micromonospora chalcea*, a whole genome sequence analysis revealed it to be most closely related to *Micromonospora tulbaghiae* 45142^T. The two strains were distinguished using a combination of genomic and phenotypic features. Based on these data, it is proposed that strain MT25^T (NCIMB 15245^T, TISTR 2834^T) be classified as *Micromonospora provocatoris* sp. nov. Analysis of the genome sequence of strain MT25^T (genome size 6.1 Mbp) revealed genes predicted to responsible for its adaptation to extreme environmental conditions that prevail in deep-sea sediments.

Keywords: Mariana Trench; *Micromonospora provocatoris* MT25; desferrioxamine; *n*-acetylglutaminyl glutamine amide; ^{1}H-^{15}N 2D-NMR; genomics; biosynthetic gene clusters; stress genes

1. Introduction

Novel filamentous actinobacteria isolated from marine sediments are a prolific source of new specialized metabolites [1–3], as exemplified by the discovery of the abyssomicins, a new family of polyketides [4] produced by *Micromonospora* (formerly *Verrucosispora*) *maris* [5] and the proximicins, novel aminofuran antibiotics and anticancer compounds isolated from *Micromonospora* (*Verrucosispora*) *fiedleri* [6,7]. Novel micromonosporae have large genomes (6.1–7.9 Mbp) which contain strain, species and clade specific biosynthetic gene clusters (BGCs) with the potential to express new bioactives [8–10] needed to counter multi-drug resistant pathogens [11]. These developments provide an objective way of prioritizing novel micromonosporae for genome mining and natural product discovery [8–10]. Key stress genes detected in the genomes of micromonosporae provide an insight into how they became adapted to harsh abiotic conditions that are characteristic of extreme biomes [8,12].

The actinobacterial genus *Micromonospora* [13] emend Nouioui et al. [5], the type genus of the family *Micromonosporaceae* [14] emend Nouioui et al. [5] is a member of the order *Micromonosporales* [15] of the class *Actinomycetia* [16]. The genus encompasses 88 validity published species (www.bacterio.net.micromonospora, accessed on 28 May 2018), including the type species *Micromonospora chalcea* [13,17]. *Micromonospora* species can be distinguished using combinations of phenotypic properties [10,18]. The application of cutting-edge taxonomic methods showed the genus to be monophyletic, clarified its subgeneric structure and provided a sound framework for the recognition of new species [5,8]. The genus typically contains aerobic to microaerophilic, Gram-positive, acid-fast-negative actinobacteria, which form single, nonmotile spores on an extensively branched substrate mycelium, lack aerial hyphae and produce either xylose or mannose or galactose and glucose as major sugars. Hydrolysates of these microorganisms are rich in *meso*- and/or dihydroxypimelic acid (A_2pm) with phosphatidylethanolamine being a diagnostic polar lipid. Iso-C15:0 and iso-C16:0 are the predominant fatty acids, while the DNA G + C percentage ranges from 65% to 75% [5,8,16].

The present study was designed to determine the taxonomic status, biotechnological potential and ecological characteristics of a *Micromonospora* strain, isolate MT25^T, recovered from sediment collected from the Challenger Deep of the Mariana Trench in the Pacific Ocean. The results of the polyphasic study together with associated genomic features showed that isolate MT25^T represents a novel species within the genus *Micromonospora* and has a large genome with the potential to express new natural products, as well as stress-related genes that provide an insight into its ability to tolerate extreme environmental conditions found in deep-sea sediments.

2. Results and Discussion

In this study we sequenced, annotated and analyzed the genome of isolate MT25^T which was recovered from sediment collected at a depth of 10,898 m from the Mariana Trench, to highlight on its taxonomic status, ability to synthesize major metabolites, as well as giving an insight into its ecological properties.

2.1. Isolation, Maintenance and Characterization of Strain MT25^T

Micromonospora strain MT25^T was isolated from a sediment sample (no. 281) taken from the Mariana Trench (Challenger Deep; 142°12′372″ E; 11°19′911″ N) using a standard dilution plate procedure [19] and raffinose-histidine agar as the selective medium [20]. The sediment was collected at a depth of 10,898 m by the remotely operated submersible Kaiko, using a sterilized mud sampler during dive 74 [21]. The sample (approximately 2 mL) was taken to the UK in an isolated container at 4 °C, then stored at −20 °C.

The strain is aerobic, Gram-positive, nonmotile, produces a branched substrate mycelium bearing single sessile spores with rugose surfaces (0.8–0.9 µm) (Figure 1 and Figure S1). Meso-A_2pm is the diamino acid of the peptidoglycan, and glucose, mannose, ribose and xylose are the major whole organism sugars. Iso-C16:0 is the predominant fatty acid, and the polar lipids are diphosphatidylglycerol, phosphatidylethanolamine (diagnostic component), phosphatidylinositol, a glycolipid and two unknown phospholipids (Figure S2). Like the other micromonosporae, the strain contains complex mixtures of saturated and unsaturated fatty acids [8,16], as shown by the presence of major proportions of iso-C16:0 (25.3% of total), anteiso-C15:OH (10.5%) and iso-C15:0 (10.0%), lower proportions of iso-C14:0 (3.6%), anteiso-C15:0 (6.9%), C16:0 (2.8%), 10-methyl C16:0 (3.0%), iso-C17:0 (4.2%), anteiso-C17:0 (8.6%), C17:1w9c (3.2%), C17:0 (3.2%), 10-methyl C17:0 (2.1%), iso-C18:0 (1.4%), C18:1w9c (3.5%), C18:0 (4.8%), 10-methyl C18:0 (1.2%) and trace amounts (<1.0%) of iso-C10:0 (0.1%), C10:0 2OH (0.1%), iso-C12:0 (0.1%), C12:0 (0.2%), iso-C13:0 (0.1%), anteiso-C13:0 (0.1%), C14:0 (0.7%), iso-C16:1 (0.6%), iso-C16:1w9c (0.6%), iso-C15:0 3OH (0.5%), anteiso-C17:1 (0.5%), iso-C17:0 3OH (0.1%) and iso-C19:0 (0.1%).

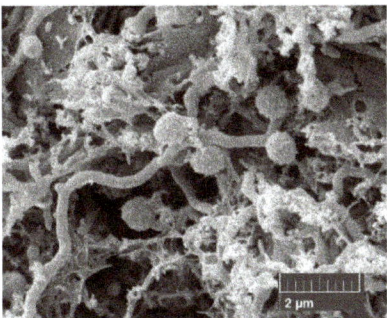

Figure 1. Scanning electron micrograph of *Micromonospora* strain MT25^T (× 2.4 k), showing the presence of single sessile spores with the rugose surfaces borne on the substrate mycelium following growth on oatmeal agar for 7 days at 28 °C.

2.2. Compound Identification

Compound **1** was obtained as a white amorphous powder, 16.2 mg; $[\alpha]_D^{25} = -47$ (c 0.1, MeOH). The IR absorption peaks of **1** suggested NH$_2$ (3408, 3326, 3316, 3274, 3230, 3202 cm^{-1}) and carbonyl groups (1670, 1660, 1655, 1647). LRESIMS measurements revealed peaks at m/z 316.1 [M + H]$^+$ and 338.1 [M + Na]$^+$ indicating that the molecular weight was 315.1. The molecular formula of **1** was established as C$_{12}$H$_{21}$N$_5$O$_5$ by HRESIMS (obsd. [M+Na]$^+$ at m/z 338.143098, calcd. for C$_{12}$H$_{21}$N$_5$O$_5$Na, 338.144046, Δ = −2.8 ppm), indicating that the molecule had five degrees of unsaturation (Figure 2).

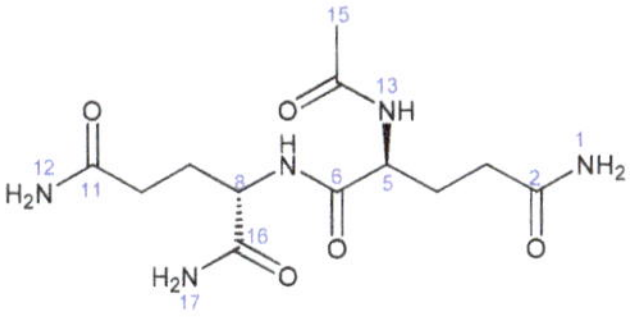

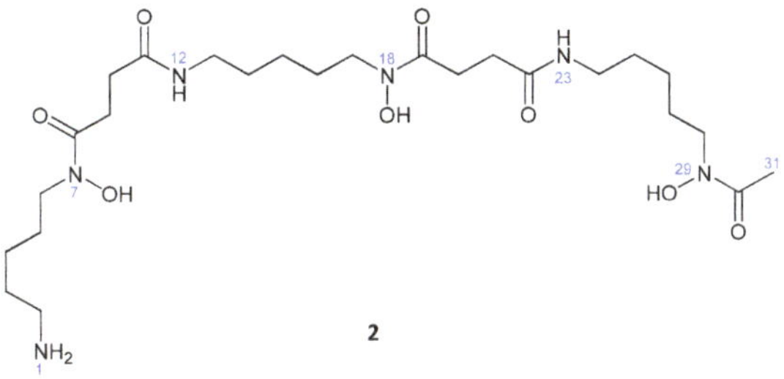

Figure 2. Chemical structures of the isolated compounds.

The 1D ^{1}H and ^{13}C NMR data (DMSO-d_6) in combination with the ^{1}H-^{13}C HSQC NMR experiments of **1** showed two methine H-5 [δ_H 4.15 (1H, m)] and H-8 [δ_H 4.12 (1H, m)]; four methylene H$_2$-10 [δ_H 2.08 (2H, m)], H$_2$-3 [δ_H 2.06 (2H, m)], H$_2$-4 [δ_H 1.89 (1H, m) and 1.74 (1H, m)], H$_2$-9 [δ_H 1.87 (1H, m) and 1.67 (1H, m)] groups and one methyl group

CH₃-15 [δ_H 1.86 (3H, s)] as well as five quaternary carbonyl carbon atoms; C-11 (δ_C 173.8 s), C-2 (δ_C 173.8 s), C-16 (δ_C 173.3 s), C-6 (δ_C 171.4 s) and C-14 (δ_C 169.7 s) (Table 1).

Table 1. ^{1}H (600 MHz), ^{13}C NMR (150 MHz) and ^{15}N (600 MHz) data (in DMSO-d_6) for compounds **1** and **2**.

No.	1			2		
	δ_C, Mult.	δ_N, Mult.	δ_H, Mult (J in Hz)	δ_C, Mult.	δ_N, Mult.	δ_H, Mult (J in Hz)
1	-	108.5, NH₂	a. 7.28, brs b. 6.75, brs	31.4 t		
2	173.8, C	-	-	41.4 t		2.76 (t, 8.0)
3	31.4, CH₂	-	2.06, m	29.2 t		1.51 m
4	27.2, CH₂	-	a. 1.89, m b. 1.74, m	25.4, t		1.38 m
5	52.7, CH	-	4.15, m	28.3 t		1.51 m
6	171.4, C	-	-	49.3 t		3.46 m
7	-	117.3, NH	7.97, d (7.8)	-	174.4, s	9.68 brs
8	52.1, CH	-	4.12, m	173.9 s		-
9	27.8, CH₂	-	a. 1.87, m b. 1.67, m	30.0 t		2.58 m
10	31.6, CH₂	-	2.08, m	31.3 t		2.27 m
11	173.8, C	-	-	173.9 s		-
12	-	108.6, NH₂	a. 7.28, brs b. 6.75, brs	-	116.2 d	7.79 brs
13	-	123.2, NH	8.11, d (7.8)	41.0 t		3.00 (q, 8.0)
14	169.7, C	-	-	31.4 t		1.38 m
15	22.6, CH₃	-	1.86, s	26.0 t		1.26 m
16	173.3, C	-	-	28.6 t		1.51 m
17	-	104.8, NH₂	a. 7.27, brs b. 7.05, brs	49.4 t		3.46 m
18				174.4 s		9.67 brs
19				173.9 s		-
20				30.1 t		2.58 m
21				32.4 t		2.27 m
22				173.9 s		-
23				-	116.2 d	7.79 brs
24				41.0 t		3.00 (q, 8.0)
25				31.4 t		1.38 m
26				26.0 t		1.26 m
27				28.6 t		1.51 m
28				49.6 t		3.46 m
29				-	175.6 s	9.63 brs
30				173.5 s		-
31				22.9 q		1.96 s

Eight hydrogen resonances lacked correlations in the ^{1}H-^{13}C HSQC 2D NMR spectrum of **1** and were therefore recognized as being located on either oxygen or nitrogen atoms. The ^{1}H-^{15}N HSQC NMR spectrum (Figure S8) of **1** indicated that all eight of these protons were bonded to nitrogen (Table 1); three as part of NH₂ groups; NH₂-17 [δ_H 7.27 (1H, brs) and 7.05 (1H, brs)], NH₂-12 [δ_H 7.28 (1H, brs) and 6.75 (1H, brs)], NH₂-1 [δ_H 7.28 (1H, brs) and 6.75 (1H, brs)] and two in NH groups; NH-13 [δ_H 8.11 (1H, d, 7.8 Hz)], NH-7 [δ_H 7.97 (1H, d, 7.8 Hz)]. Also, from the ^{1}H-^{15}N HSQC and the ^{1}H-^{15}N HMBC 2D-NMR spectra (DMSO-d_6) of **1** it was possible to assign the resonance of each nitrogen; NH-13 (δ_N 123.2 t), NH-7 (δ_N 117.3 d), NH₂-12 (δ_N 108.6 t), NH₂-17 (δ_N 104.8 t) and NH₂-1 (δ_N 108.5 t) (Figure 3 and Figure S8).

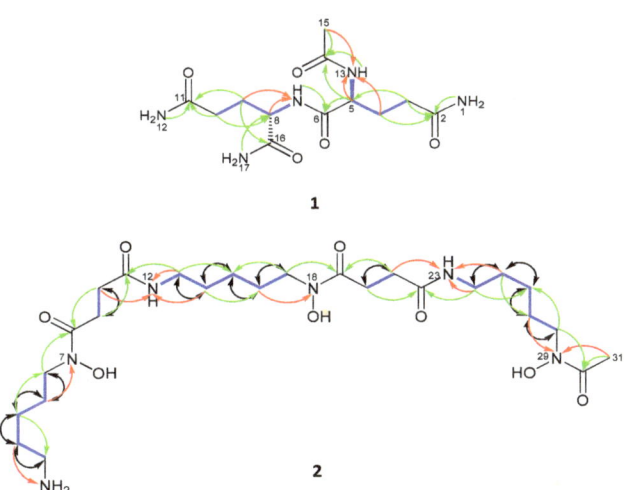

Figure 3. Selected COSY (blue), ^{1}H-^{13}C HMBC (H→C) (green), ^{1}H-^{15}N HMBC (H→N) (red) and 1,1-ADEQUATE (H→C) (black) correlations.

With all protons assigned to their directly bonded carbon and nitrogen atoms it was possible to deduce substructures with the aid of the ^{1}H-^{1}H COSY spectrum of **1** (Figure 3). The connectivities between substructures were established from key ^{1}H-^{13}C HMBC correlations (Figure 3). Thus, correlations between C-2 (δ_C 173.8) and H$_2$-3, H$_2$-1 and between C-11 (δ_C 173.8) and H$_2$-10, H$_2$-12 as well as between C-5 (δ_C 52.7) and H$_2$-3 and between C-8 (δ_C 52.1) and H$_2$-17 and between C-14 (δ_C 169.7) and H-5, H-13, H$_3$-15 and between C-16 and H-8, H$_2$-9 and H$_2$-17 clearly defined the planar structure as shown in **1**. Finally, the positions of nitrogen were defined from ^{1}H-^{15}N-HMBC which showed long range correlations between N-13 and H4a/b and H3-15 and between N-7 and H9a/b (Figure 3 and Figure S9). Given these results and comparisons with previously data [22], the compound was identified as *n*-acetylglutaminyl glutamine amide.

Compound **2** was identified as deferoxamine B. Its molecular formula was established as $C_{25}H_{49}N_6O_8$ by HRESIMS (*m/z* 561.3577 [M + H]$^+$, calcd. for $C_{25}H_{49}N_6O_8$, 561.3592, Δ = −2.6 ppm), which required five degrees of unsaturation, and also found bound to Fe^{+3} (*m/z* 614.2780 [M + Fe − 2H]$^+$) (Figure 2).

The full planar structure of **2** was assigned by interpretation of 1D (^{1}H and ^{13}C) in connection with extensive 2D-NMR (^{1}H-^{1}H COSY, ^{1}H-^{13}C HSQC, ^{1}H-^{13}C HMBC, HSQC-TOCSY and 1,1-ADEQUATE) spectroscopic data recorded in (DMSO-d_6) (Table 1), and by comparing it with the previously reported data on desferrioxamine [23].

The 1D ^{1}H and ^{13}C NMR spectra (DMSO-d_6) in combination with ^{1}H-^{13}C HSQC experiments of **2** exhibited the presence of 31 carbons, including: one methyl CH$_3$-31[(δ_H 2.14 (3H s), (δ_C 21.9 q)], nineteen methylenes grouped by interpretation of ^{1}H-^{1}H COSY and 1,1-ADEQUATE experiments into five spin systems, including: H$_2$-2 to H$_2$-6; H$_2$-9 and H$_2$-10; H$_2$-13 to H$_2$-17; H$_2$-20 and H$_2$-21; H$_2$-24 to H$_2$-28 and five quaternary carbonyl carbons C-8 (δ_C 173.9 s), C-11 (δ_C 174.7 s), C-19 (δ_C 173.9 s), C-22 (δ_C 174.9 s) and C-30 (δ_C 173.8 s).

Seven hydrogen resonances lacked correlations in the ^{1}H-^{13}C HSQC spectrum of **2** and were therefore recognized as being located on either oxygen or nitrogen. From the results of a ^{1}H-^{15}N HSQC measurement made with **2** it was evident that four protons were bonded to nitrogen: comprising one NH$_2$ group; NH$_2$-1 and two NH groups; NH-12 [δ_H 7.79 (1H, brs)] and NH-23 [δ_H 7.79 (1H, brs)]. Also, from the ^{1}H-^{15}N HSQC and ^{1}H-^{15}N HMBC 2D-NMR spectra of **2** (Figure 3) it was possible to assign the resonance of each nitrogen: NH$_2$-1 (δ_N 31.4 t), NH-12 (δ_N 116.2 d), NH-23 (δ_N 116.2 d), N-7 (δ_N 174.4 s), N-18 (δ_N 174.4 s) and N-29 (δ_N 175.6 s).

With all protons assigned to their directly bonded carbon and nitrogen atoms it was possible to deduce substructures. The connectivities between these substructures were established from key ^{1}H-^{13}C HMBC and ^{1}H-^{15}N HMBC correlations (Figure 3 and Figure S21). The positions of nitrogen in amide formation were confirmed by ^{15}N-HMBC that showed correlation from H-3 to NH$_2$-1; H-5 to N-7; H-10, H-13 and H-14 to NH-12; H-16 to N-18; H-21, H-24 and H-25 to NH-23 and H-27 and H-31 to N-29 (Figure S21). The 1,1-ADEQUATE experiment confirmed the correlations of ^{1}H-^{1}H COSY and partial substructures through its two bond correlations (Figure 3 and Figure S23). The 1,1-ADEQUATE is a technique used to obtain heteronuclear correlations similarly to ^{1}H-^{13}C HMBC. While correlation signals from HMBC do not separate $^2J_{CH}$ from $^3J_{CH}$, 1,1-adequate, which exclusively observes $^1J_{CH}$ and $^2J_{CH}$, and can be combined with ^{1}H-^{13}C HSQC to identify $^2J_{CH}$. Interpretation of HSQC-TOCSY confirmed the spin systems via correlations from H-7, H-6, H-5, H-4, H-3 to C-2; H-9 to C-10; NH-12, H-14, H-15, H-16, H-17 to C-13; H-20 to C-21 and NH-23, H-25, H-26, H-27, H-28 to C-24 and confirmed the full structure of desferrioxamine B (2).

2.3. Genome Sequencing and Annotation

The whole genome sequencing reads of strain MT25^T, generated using an Ion Torrent PGM instrument, 316v2 chips and Ian on PGM Hi-QTM View Sequencing Kit, were assembled using the Ion Torrent SPAdes plugin (v. 5.0.0.0) program (Life Technologies Limited, Paisley, UK). The size of whole genome sequence of the strain represented by 1170 contigs is 6,053,796 bp with a G + C content of 71.6%. Additional genomic features of the strain are shown in Table 2 according to GenBank NCBI prokaryotic genome annotation pipeline [24–26].

Table 2. Genomic features of *Micromonospora* strain MT25^T.

Features	Strain MT25^T
Assembly size, bp	6,053,796
No. of contigs	1170
G + C (%)	71.6
Fold coverage	39.94×
N50	8214
L50	203
Genes	6643
CDs	6573
Pseudo genes	2188
Protein encoding genes	4385
rRNA	8
tRNA	59
ncRNAs	3
Accession No.	NZ_QNTW00000000
Assembly method	SPAdes v. 5.0.0.0

2.4. Phylogeny

The phylogenetic tree (Figure 4) based on almost complete 16S rRNA gene sequences shows that *Micromonospora* strain MT25^T belongs to a well-supported lineage together with the type strains of nine *Micromonospora* species. It is most closely related to *M. chalcea* DSM 43026^T. With only 4 nucleotides difference within a 1437 sequence, the 16S rRNA sequences of these two strains are 99.7% identical. The 16S rRNA of strain MT25^T also shares a relatively high sequence identify with the *Micromonospora aurantiaca* [27], *Micromonospora marina* [28], *Micromonospora maritima* [29], *Micromonospora sediminicola* [30] and *Micromonospora tulbaghiae* [31,32] strains. The close relationship between these species is in a good agreement with the results from previous 16S rRNA gene sequence analyses [8,33].

The sequence similarities between the 16S rRNA sequences of strain MT25^T and the other *Micromonospora* strains range from 88.6 to 99.1%, which is equivalent to 13 to 20 nucleotide differences.

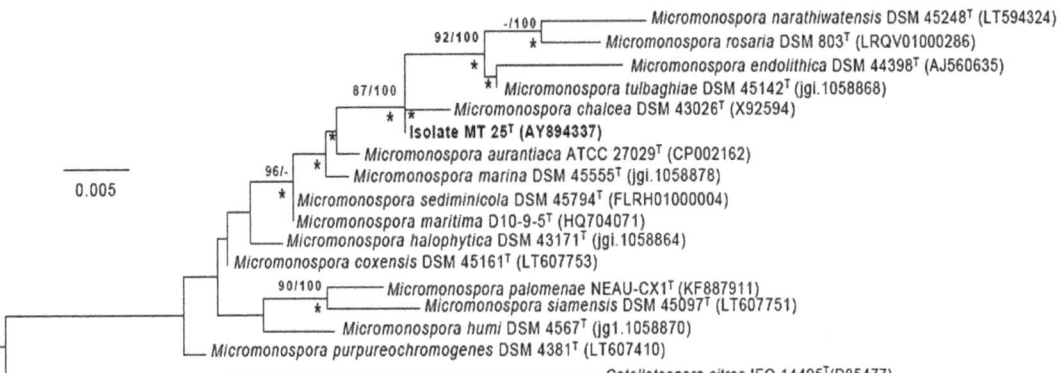

Figure 4. Maximum-likelihood tree based on almost complete 16S rRNA gene sequences generated using the GTR-GAMMA model showing relationships between isolate MT25^T and the type strains of the closest phylogenetic neighbors. Asterisks indicate branches of the tree that were also formed using the maximum-parsimony and neighbor-forming algorithms. The numbers at the nodes are bootstrap support values greater than 60% for ML (left) and MP (right). The root of the tree was established using *Catellatospora citrea* IFO 14495^T. The scale bar indicates 0.005 substitutions per nucleotide position.

Greater confidence can be placed in the topology of phylogenetic trees based on whole genome sequences than on corresponding 16S rRNA gene trees, as the former are generated from millions, as opposed to hundreds, of unit characters [5]. The phylogenomic tree (Figure 5) shows that the strain MT25^T is most closely related to *M. tulbaghiae* DSM 45124^T. In turn, these strains belong to a well-supported lineage which includes the *M. aurantiaca, M. chalcea, M. marina, M. maritima* and *M. sediminicola* strains together with the type strain of *M. humi* [34], all of these species belong to a distinct taxon, group 1a, highlighted in the genome-based classification of the genus *Micromonospora* generated by Carro et al. [8].

The recommended thresholds used to distinguish between closely related prokaryotic species based on average nucleotide identity (ANI) and digital DNA-DNA hybridization (dDDH) values are 95 to 96% [35,36] and 70% [36,37], respectively. Table 3 shows that the ANI and dDDH similarities between strain MT25^T and *M. aurantiaca* ATCC 27029^T, *M. chalcea* DSM 43026^T and *M. marina* DSM 45555^T, its three closest phylogenomic neighbors, are below the cut-off points used to assign closely related strains to the same species. The ANI and dDDH values also provide further evidence that strain MT25^T is most closely related to *M. tulbaghiae* DSM 45142^T. However, the relationship between these strains is not clear-cut as they share a dDDH value below the 70% threshold and an ANI value at the borderline used to assign closely related strains to the same species. Conflicting results such as these are not unusual, as exemplified by studies on closely related *Micromonospora* and *Rhodococcus* species [33,38]. In such instances, ANI and dDDH similarities need to be interpreted with a level of flexibility and should also be seen within the context of other biological features, such ecological, genomic and phenotypic criteria [33,38,39]. Again, the use of a universal ANI threshold for the delineation of prokaryotic species has been questioned [40].

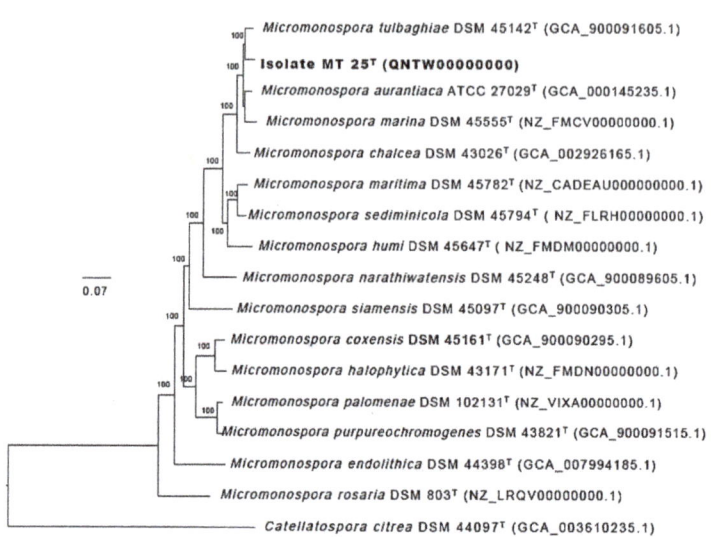

Figure 5. Maximum-likelihood phylogenomic tree based on 704 single copy core genes showing relationships between isolate MT25^T and closely related type strains of *Micromonospora* species. Numbers at the nodes are bootstrap support values based on 100 replicates. GenBank accession numbers are shown in parentheses. The scale bar indicates 0.07 substitutions per nucleotide position. The tree is rooted using the type strain of *Catellatospora citrea*.

Table 3. Average nucleotide identity (ANI) and digital DNA-DNA hybridization (dDDH) similarities between *Micromonospora* strain MT25^T and its closest phylogenomic neighbors.

Phylogenomic Neighbors	Similarity ANI	Values (%) dDDH
M. aurantiaca ATCC 27029^T	95.2	62.7
M. chalcea DSM 43026^T	93.5	53.0
M. marina DSM 45555^T	94.6	58.6
M. tulbaghiae DSM 45142^T	96.0	68.1

2.5. Species Assignment

It can be seen from Table 4 that strain MT25^T and *M. tulbaghiae* DSM 45142^T, its closest phylogenomic neighbor, have phenotypic features in common though a range of other properties can be weighted to distinguish between them. Strain MT25^T, unlike the *M. tulbaghiae* strain, grows at pH 6 and 10, reduces nitrate and shows much greater activity in the AP1-ZYM tests. In contrast, the *M. tulbaghiae* strain, unlike strain MT25^T, grows at 4 °C, in the presence of 5% w/v sodium chloride, produces hydrogen sulfide and shows greater activity in the degradation tests. In addition, strain MT25^T produces sessile, rugose ornamental single spores on the substrate mycelium (Figure 1) whereas the *M. tulbaghiae* strain bears smooth, single spores borne on sporophores [31]. Further, strain MT25^T produces an orange as opposed to a brown substrate mycelium on yeast-malt extract agar though the colonies of both strains become dark brown/black on sporulation. The two strains also have different cellular sugar profiles as only strain MT25^T produces mannose. They can also be distinguished using a range of genomic features, notably genome size and G + C content. The genome size of strain MT25^T is 6.05 Mbp and its G + C content is 71.6%, whilst the corresponding figures for the *M. tulbaghiae* strain are 6.5 Mbp and 73.0%. Genome size and G + C content are considered to be conserved within species and can therefore represent useful taxonomic markers [5]. Inter-species variation in genomic G + C content does not usually exceed 1% [5,41].

Table 4. Phenotypic properties that distinguish isolate MT25^T from *M. tulbaghiae* DSM 45142^T.

Characteristics	Strain MT25^T	*M. tulbaghiae* DSM 45142^T
Morphology:		
Spores borne on sporophores	-	+
Spore ornamentation	Rugose	Smooth
Substrate mycelial color on yeast extract-malt extract agar	Orange	Brown
AP1-ZYM tests:		
Acid and alkaline phosphatases, β-glucosidase, lipase (C14), naphthol-AS-BI-phosphohydrolase	+	-
α-galacosidase, β-glucoronidase, N-acetyl-β-glucosaminidase	-	+
Biochemical tests:		
H$_2$S production	-	+
Nitrate reduction	+	-
Degradation tests:		
L-tyrosine	+	-
Casein	-	+
Gelatin	-	+
Starch	-	+
Tween-80	-	+
Tolerance tests:		
Growth at 4 °C	-	+
Growth at pH 6.0 and pH 10	+	-
Growth in presence of 5% *w/v* NaCl	-	+
Chemotaxonomy:		
Major whole-organism sugars	Glucose, mannose, ribose and xylose	Glucose, ribose and xylose

+, positive results; -, negative results. * Data for the biochemical, chemotaxonomic, tolerance and morphological properties on the *M. tulbaghiae* DSM 45142^T were taken from Kirby and Meyer (2010) [31]. Each strain grew from 10 to 37 °C, from pH 7 to 9, and were positive for α-chymotrypsin, cystine and valine arylamidases, esterase (C4), esterase lipase (C8), β-galactosidase and trypsin, but negative for α-fucosidase, α-mannosidase and β-glucoronidase. Neither strain degraded xylan.

In light of all of these data, it can be concluded that although strains MT25^T and *M. tulbaghiae* DSM 45142^T are close phylogenomic neighbors which can be distinguished using a combination of genomic and phenotypic properties, notably their genome sizes and G+C contents. It is, therefore, proposed that isolate MT25^T be considered as the type strain of a novel *Micromonospora* species that belongs to the phylogenomic group 1a, as designed by Carro et al. [8]. The name proposed for this species is *Micromonospora provocatoris* sp. nov.

2.6. Description of Micromonospora provocatoris sp. nov.

Micromonospora provocatoris (pro.vo.ca.to'ris. L. gen. n. *provocatoris*, of a challenger, referring to the Challenger Deep of the Mariana Trench, the source of the isolate), Aerobic, Gram-positive strain, non-acid-fast actinobacterium which forms nonmotile, single, sessile spores (0.8–0.9 μm) with rugose ornamentation on extensively branched substrate hyphae, but does not produce aerial hyphae. Colonies are orange on oatmeal agar eventually turning black on sporulation (Figure S2). Growth Occurs between pH 6.0 and 8.0, optimally at pH 7.0, from 10 °C to 37 °C, optimally at 28 °C and in the presence of 1% *w/v* sodium chloride. Aesculin is hydrolyzed and catalase produced. Degrades arbutin and L-tyrosine, but not starch or xylan. Furthermore, acid and alkaline phosphatases, α-chymotrypsin, cystine, leucine and valine arylamidases, esterase (C4), lipase esterase (C8), lipase (C14), β-galactosidase, β-glucosidase, naphthol-AS-BI-phosphohydrolase and trypsin are produced, but not α-fucosidase, α-galacturonidase, β-glucuronidase or α-mannosidase. The cell wall contains *meso*-A$_2$pm, and the whole cell sugars are glucose, mannose, ribose and xylose. The predominant fatty acid is iso-C16:0 and the polar lipid profile contains diphosphatidylglycerol, phosphatidylethanolamine and phosphatidylinositol, a glycolipid and two unidentified phospholipids. The dDNA G + C content of the type and only strain is 71.6% and it is genome size 6.05 Mbp.

The type strain MT25^T (= NCIMB 15245^T = TISTR 2834^T) was isolated from surface sediment from the Challenger Deep in the Mariana Trench of the Pacific Ocean. The accession numbers of the 16S rRNA gene sequence and that of the whole genome of the strain are AY894337 and QNTW00000000, respectively.

2.7. Specialised Metabolite-Biosynthetic Gene Clusters

Antibiotic and Secondary Metabolites Analysis Shell "AntiSMASH 6.0.0 0 alpha 1" [42] predicts natural products-biosynthetic gene clusters (NP-BGCs) that are based on the percentage of genes from the closest known bioclusters which share BLAST hits to the genome of the strains under consideration. Mining the draft genome of *M. provocatoris* MT25^T revealed the presence of ten known BGCs (Table 5). Two gene clusters were predicted to be responsible for the biosynthesis of siderophore desferrioxamine B, which was initially isolated from *Streptomyces* strain 1D38640 [43], and rhizomide A, which has antitumor and antimicrobial properties [44]. The other gene clusters found are likely to be involved with the biosynthesis of such products as phosphonoglycans, alkyl-O-dihydrogeranyl-methoxyhydroquinones [45], and the antibiotics kanamycin [46], brasilicardin A and frankiamicin [47,48]. Interestingly, two bioclusters belonging to two classes I lanthipeptides and a class III lanthipeptide lacked any homology thereby providing further evidence that NP-BGCs are discontinuously distributed in the genomes of *Micromonospora* taxa [8,9].

Table 5. Identity of predicted natural product biosynthetic gene clusters using antiSMASH 6.0.0 alpha 1.

BGCs	No.	Nucleotide (nt) bp	Type	Accession Number	Homologue	Accession Number	Identity
Siderophore	1	6963	Desferrioxamine E	QNTW01000257	Desferrioxamine EBGC from *Streptomyces* sp. ID38640	MG459167.1	100%
T2PKS *	1	3695	Frankiamicin	QNTW01000523	Frankiamicin BGC from *Frankia* sp. EAN1pec	CP000820.1	28%
Terpene	1	20066	Isorenieratene	QNTW01000028	Isorenieratene BGC from *Streptomyces griseus* subsp. *griseus* NBRC 13350	AP009493.1	28%
Terpene	1	11057	Phosphonoglycans	QNTW01000118	Phosphonoglycans BGC from *Glycomyces* sp. NRRL B-16210	KJ125437.1	3%
Oligosaccharides	1		Brasilicardin A		Brasilicardin A BGC from *Nocardia terpenica* IFM 0406	KV411304.1	23%
NRPS ***	1	10526	Rhizomide (A-C)	QNTW01000131	Rhizomide A BGC from *Paraburkholderia rhizoxinica* HKI 454	NC_014718.1	100%
T3PKS **	1	12,601	Alkyl-O-dihydrogeranyl-methoxyhydroquinones	QNTW01000093	alkyl-O-dihydrogeranyl-methoxyhydroquinones biosynthetic gene cluster from *Actinoplanes missouriensis* 431	AP012319.1	28%
Lanthipeptide-class-i	1	26,371	Kanamycin	QNTW01000003	kanamycin biosynthetic gene cluster from *Streptomyces kanamyceticus*	AB254080.1	1%
Lanthipeptide-class-i	1	18,770	No match found	QNTW01000004	-	-	-
Lanthipeptide-class-iii	1	7750	No match found	QNTW01000229	-	-	-

* Type II and III PKS cluster, ** Type III PKS cluster and *** Non-ribosomal peptide synthetase cluster.

2.8. Genes Potentially Associated with Enviromental Stress

Stress-related genes detected in the genome of *Dermacoccus abyssi* strain MT1.1^T, an isolate from the same sediment sample as the *M. provocatoris* strain, gave clues to how this piezotolerant strain became adapted to environmental conditions which prevail in sea-floor sediment of the Challenger Deep of the Mariana Trench [49]. In the present study, the genome of *M. provocatoris* strain MT25^T annotated using NCBI Genbank [24–26] pipeline was seen to harbor genes associated with a range of stress responses, notably ones linked with carbon starvation, cold shock response, high pressure, osmoregulation and oxidative stress (Table S3), as was the case with the *D. abyssi* strain.

Deep-sea psychrophilic bacteria synthesize cold shock proteins essential for adaptation to low temperatures [50–52]. The genome of strain MT25^T contained genes predicted to encode cold shock proteins, as exemplified by genes *clpB* and *hscB* which are associated with the synthesis of ATP-dependent and Fe-S chaperones, respectively [52–54]. The genome also contains gene *deaD* encoding an RNA helicase involved in cold shock response and adaptation [55]. The strain has genes associated with the synthesis of branch-chain and long chain polysaturated fatty acids that are linked to membrane fluidity and functionality at low temperatures [49,52], including *fabF*, *fabG*, *fabH* and *fabI* genes which are responsible for the biosynthesis of β-ketoacyl-ACP synthase II, 3-oxoacyl-ACP reductase, ketoacyl-ACP synthase III, enoyl-ACP reductase and enoyl-ACP reductase, respectively (Table S3). The synthesis of low-melting point branched-chain and/or polyunsaturated fatty acids (PUFAs) is crucial as it allows organisms in cold environments to maintain membrane fluidity in a liquid crystalline state thereby allowing organisms to resist freeze-thaw cycles at low temperatures [56,57]. Low temperatures reduce enzymatic activity leading to the generation of reactive oxygen species (ROS). The genome of strain MT25^T contains genes *sodN*, *trxA* and *trxB* predicted to encode products that offset the harmful effects of superoxide dismutase, thioredoxin and thioredoxin-disulfide reductase respectively.

Bacteria living in deep-sea habitats have developed ways of dealing with osmotic stress, notably by synthesizing osmoregulators, these are small organic molecules (compatible solutes) induced under hyperosmotic stress [58–60]. In this context, strain MT25^T contains genes predicted to be involved in the biosynthesis of compatible solutes, such as *opuA* gene, which regulates the uptake of glycine/betaine thereby contributing to osmotic stress responses [61,62]. Similarly, genes *asnO* and *ngg* are predicted to be involved in the production of osmoprotectant NAGGN (*n*-acetylglutaminylglutamine amide) that has an important role in counteracting osmotic stress in deep-sea environments. It is produced by many bacteria grown at high osmolarity bacteria, such as *Sinorhizobium meliloti* [63].

Another consequence of high pressure on bacteria is that the transport of compounds, such as amino acids, is reduced leading to upregulation of transported molecules [64]. Genes associated with the production of different types of ABC transporter permeases were detected in strain MT25^T including branched-chain amino acid permeases that are upregulated at high pressure [65]. In addition, the genome of strain MT25^T contains pressure sensing and pressure adaptation genes, as illustrated by *cycD*, *mdh* and *asd* genes, which are linked to the production of a thiol reductant ABC exporter subunit, malate dehydrogenase and aspartate semialdehyde dehydrogenase, respectively. Similarly, *secD* and *secF* are predicted to encode protein translocase subunits and *secG* preprotein translocase unit [65,66], as shown in Table S3.

Bacteria able to grow in nutrient-limiting conditions need to store carbon compounds like glycogen [67]. In this respect, it is interesting that strain MT25^T contains a gene, *gigA*, which is predicted to encode glycogen synthase and another gene, *gigx*, which is linked with the production of a glycogen debranching enzyme responsible for the breakdown of this storage molecule. Furthermore, the strain has the capacity to produce carbonic anhydrase proteins which are required for fixation of carbon dioxide [65,68] thereby suggesting that its potential to grow as a lithoautotroph. This discovery provides further evidence that filamentous actinobacteria in carbon-limiting, extreme biomes are capable of adopting a lithoautotrophic lifestyle, as shown by the type strains of novel *Blastococcus*, *Geodermatophilus* and *Modestobacter* species [69–73].

Micromonosporae can grow under aerobic and microaerophilic conditions. Their ability to tolerate low oxygen tensions indicates an ability to grow in oxygen depleted biomes, such as lake and river sediments and soil prone to flooding [74,75]. Genome mining of strain MT25^T revealed many putative genes predicted to encode terminal oxidases involved in aerobic respiration, as witnessed by the *cydB* gene encoding cytochrome *d* ubiquinol oxidase subunit II, and genes *ctad* and *coxb* expressing cytochrome *c* oxidase subunits I and II, respectively. Several terminal dehydrogenase and reductase encoding genes involved in respiratory chains were detected, including ones predicted to express arsenate reductase *arsc* and ferredoxin reductase. Multiple genes predicted to encode succinate dehydrogenase used as electron donors under low oxygen conditions were also detected in the genome of strain MT25^T. Further support for the ability of the strain to adapt to different oxygen levels reflects its capacity to form cytochrome oxidase complexes that have different affinities for oxygen. Biological adaptations such as these may account for the presence of micromonosporae (including verrucosisporae) in marine habitats, including deep-sea sediments [2,3,76].

3. Materials and Methods

3.1. Microorganism

Micromonospora strain MT25^T was isolated from Mariana Trench sediment, sample no. 281, collected at a depth of 10,898 m (Challenger Deep; 11°19′911″ N; 142°12′372″ E) by the remotely operated submersible Kaiko, using a sterilized mud sampler, on 21 May 1998, during dive number 74. The sample was transported to the UK in an insulated container at 4 °C and stored at −20 °C until examined for actinobacteria. The test strain was isolated, purified and maintained using procedures described by Pathom-aree et al. [19]. *M. tulbaghiae* DSM 45142^T was maintained under the same conditions.

3.2. General Experimental Procedures

General Experimental Procedures. ^{1}H, ^{13}C, ^{15}N NMR experiments were recorded on a Bruker Avance 600 MHz NMR spectrometer AVANCE III HD (Billerica, MA, USA) equipped with a cryoprobe, in DMSO-d_6. Low resolution electrospray mass spectra were obtained using a Perseptive Biosystems Mariner LC-MS (PerSeptive Biosystems, Framingham, MA, USA), and high-resolution mass data were generated on Finnigan MAT 900 XLT (Thermo-Finnigan, San Jose, CA, USA). HPLC separations were carried out using a Phenomenex reversed-phase (C_{18}, 10 Å × 10 mm × 250 mm) column and an Agilent 1100 series gradient pump and monitored using an Agilent DAD G1315B variable-wavelength UV detector (Agilent Technologies, Waldbronn, Germany).

3.3. Fermentation Conditions

For the first-stage seed preparation, an agar grown culture of strain MT25^T, was inoculated into 10 mL of GYE medium (4.0 g glucose, 4.0 g yeast extract, agar 15 g, distilled H_2O 1 L, pH 7.0). After 5 days incubation at 28 °C, with agitation, the first stage culture was used to inoculate the production fermentation, using ISP2 broth (yeast extract 4 g, malt extract 10 g, glucose 4 g, $CaCO_3$ 2 g, distilled H_2O 1 L, pH 7.3). The fermentation was incubated at 28 °C, with agitation, and the biomass was harvested on the seventh day. All media components were purchased from Sigma-Aldrich (St. Louis, MO, USA).

3.4. Isolation and Purification of Secondary Metabolites

Harvested fermentation broth (6 L) was centrifuged at 3000 rpm for 20 min, and the HP20 resin together with the cell mass was washed with distilled water then extracted with MeOH (3 × 500 mL). The MeOH extracts were combined and concentrated under reduced pressure to yield 6.39 g solid extract. The extract was suspended in 250 mL of MeOH and then partitioned with *n*-hexane (3 × 250 mL). The remaining MeOH solubles were the subject of further purification by Sephadex LH-20 column chromatography (CH$_2$Cl$_2$/MeOH 1:1) to yield 3 fractions. Final purification was achieved using reversed–phase HPLC (C$_{18}$, 10 µm, 10 mm × 250 mm), employing gradient elution from 0–90% CH$_3$CN/H$_2$O containing 0.01% TFA over 40 min for fraction A (23 mg) to give compound **1** (16.2 mg) and fraction B (27 mg) and to give compound **2** (9.4 mg).

Compound (**1**): white amorphous powder, 16.2 mg; $[\alpha]_D^{25} = -47$ (c 0.1, MeOH); IR ν_{max}: 3408, 3326, 3316, 3274, 3230, 3202, 1670, 1660, 1655, 1647, 1445, 1237 cm^{-1}; LRESIMS m/z 338.10 [M + Na]$^+$; HRESIMS m/z 338.143098 [M + Na]$^+$ (calcd for C$_{12}$H$_{21}$N$_5$O$_5$Na, 338.144046, $\Delta = -2.8$ ppm).; ^{1}H and ^{13}C NMR data (DMSO-d_6), see Table 1.

Compound (**2**): colorless amorphous substance, 9.4 mg; IR ν_{max}: 3315, 3090, 2860, 1625, 1560, 1460, 1270, 1225, 1190 cm^{-1}; HRESIMS m/z 561.3577 [M + H]$^+$ (calcd for C$_{25}$H$_{49}$N$_6$O$_8$, 561.3592, $\Delta = -2.6$ ppm).; ^{1}H and ^{13}C NMR data (DMSO-d_6), see Table 1.

3.5. Phylogeny

An almost complete 16S rRNA gene sequence (1437 nucleotides) (Genbank accession number AY894337) was taken directly from the draft genome of the isolate using the ContEst16S tool from the EzBioCloud webserver (https://www.ezbiocloud.net/tools/contest16s, accessed on 1 June 2018) [77]. The sequence was aligned with corresponding sequences of the most closely related type strains of *Micromonospora* species drawn from the EzBioCloud webserver [78] using MUSCLE software (Version No. 3.8.31, drive5, Berkeley, CA, USA) [79]. Pairwise sequence similarities were generated using the single gene tree option from the Genome-to-Genome Distance calculator (GGDC) webserver [37,80] and phylogenetic trees inferred using the maximum-likelihood [81], maximum-parsimony [82] and neighbor-joining [83] algorithms. A ML (maximum likelihood) tree was generated from alignments with RAxML (Randomized Axelerated Maximum Likelihood) [84] using rapid bootstrapping with the auto Maximum-Relative-Error (MRE) criterion [85] and a MP tree inferred from alignments with the tree analysis using the New Technology (TNT) program [86] with 1000 bootstraps together with tree-bisection-and-reconnection branch swapping and ten random sequence addition replicates. The sequences were checked for computational bias using the x_2 test taken from PAUP * (Phylogenetic analysis using parsimony) [87]. The trees were evaluated using bootstrap analyses based on 1000 replicates [88] from the MEGA X software package (Version No. 10.0.5, MEGA development team, State College, PA, USA) [89] and the two-parameter model of Jukes and Cantor, 1969 [90]. The 16S rRNA gene sequence of *Catellatospora citrea* IFO 14495^T (D85477) was used to root the tree.

3.6. Phenotypic Characterisation

The isolate was examined for a broad range of phenotype properties known to be of value in *Micromonospora* systematics [10,16]. Standard chromatographic procedures were used to detect isomers of diaminopimelic acid [91], whole-organism sugars [92] and polar lipids [93,94], using freeze dried biomass harvested from yeast extract-malt extract broth cultures (International Streptomyces Project [ISP] medium 2) [95]. Similarly, cellular fatty acids extracted from the isolate were methylated and analyzed using the Sherlock Microbial Identification (MIDI) system and the resultant peaks identified using the ACTINO 6 database [96].

Cultural and morphological properties of the isolate were recorded following growth on oatmeal agar (ISP medium 3) [95]. Growth from the oatmeal agar plate was examined for micromorphological traits using a scanning electron microscope (Tescan Vega 3, LMU instrument, Fuveau, France) and the protocol described by O'Donnell et al. [97]. The enzymatic profiles of strain MT25^T and M. tulbaghiae DSM 45142^T were determined using AP1-ZYM strips (bioMérieux) by following the instructions of the manufacture. Similarly, biochemical, degradation, physiological and staining properties were acquired using media and methods described by Williams et al. [98]. The ability of strain MT25^T to grow under different temperature and pH regimes and in the presence of various concentrations of sodium chloride were recorded on ISP2 agar as the basal medium; the pH values were determined using phosphate buffers. All of these tests were carried out using a standard inoculum of spores and mycelial fragments equivalent to 5.0 on the McFarland scale [99].

3.7. Whole-Genome Sequencing

3.7.1. DNA Extraction and Genome Sequencing

Genomic DNA was extracted from wet biomass of a single colony of strain MT25^T following growth on yeast extract-malt extract agar for 7 days at 28 °C [95], using the modified CTAB method [100]. The sequence library was prepared using a NEB Next Fast DNA Fragmentation and Library Preparation Kit for an Ion Torrent (New England Biolabs, Hitchin, UK).

Briefly, the DNA sample (0.5 µg) was subjected to enzymatic fragmentation, end repaired and ligated to A1 and P2 adapters, followed by extraction of 490–500 bp fragments and PCR amplification. The PCR products were analyzed using a High Sensitivity DNA kit and BioAnalyser 2100 (Agilent Technologies LDA).

(UK Limited, Cheshire, UK). AMPure XP beads (Beckman Coulter, Brea, CA, USA) were used for DNA purification according to the protocol. The library was diluted to give a final concentration of 25 pM, and a template was prepared using an Ion PGM Hi-Q™ (Life Technologies Limited, Paisley, UK) View OT2 Kit and IonTorrent One Touch system OT2. The recovery of positive Ion Sphere Particles was achieved using the One Touch ES enrichment system. The sequencing reaction was conducted using an Ion PGM Hi-Q™ View Sequencing Kit, 316v2 chips and an IonTorrent PGM instrument with 850 sequencing flows, according to manufacturer's instructions (Life Technologies Limited, Paisley, UK), required for 400 nt read lengths.

3.7.2. Annotation of Genome and Bioinformatics

The sequencing reads were mapped onto reference genome sequences using CLC Genomics Workbench software (GWB, ver. 7.5, QIAGEN, LLC, Germantown, MD, USA). The reads were assembled using SPAdes v. 5.0.0.0 plugin (LifeTechnologies, Thermo Fisher Scientific, UK). The annotation of the genomic sequence was performed via NCBI GenBank annotation pipeline [24,101].

3.7.3. Detection of the Gene Clusters

The whole genome sequence of strain MT25^T was mined using AntiSMASH 6.0.0 alpha 1 ("Antibiotic and Secondary Metabolites Analysis Shell") [42] to detect biosynthetic gene clusters. The NCBI [24–26] GenBank annotation pipeline was used to detect the genes and proteins associated with bacterial adaptation.

3.7.4. GenBank Accession Number

This Whole Genome Shotgun sequence has been deposited at DDBJ/ENA/GenBank under accession number NZ_QNTW00000000. The version described in this paper is NZ_QNTW00000000.1.

3.8. Comparison of Genomes

The draft genome sequence of strain MT25^T was compared with corresponding sequences of the type strains of closely related *Micromonospora* strains, as shown in the phylogenomic analyses. A ML phylogenomic tree inferred using the codon tree option in the PATRIC webserver [102], based on aligned amino acids and nucleotides derived from 704 single copy core genes in the genome dataset matched against the PATRIC PGFams database (http://www.patricbrc.org, accessed on 10 July 2018), was generated using the RAxML algorithm [84]. Average nucleotide identity (ortho ANI) [103] and digital DNA-DNA hybridization [38] values were determined between the isolate and the type strains of *M. aurantiaca*, *M. chalcea*, *M. marina* and *M. tulbaghiae*, its closest phylogenomic neighbors.

4. Conclusions

Micromonospora strain MT25^T, an isolate recovered from sediment taken from the Mariana Trench in the Pacific Ocean, was shown to be most closely related to the type strain *M. tulbaghiae* following a genome-based classification. Characterization of strain MT25^T using a range of methods suggests that it belongs to a new *Micromonospora* species, which we name as *Micromonospora provocatoris* sp. nov. An associated bioassay-guided study together with structural analyses showed that the isolate has a potential to synthesize two major metabolites, *n*-acetylglutaminyl glutamine amide and desferrioxamine B. In line with previous studies on micromonosporae isolated from extreme habitats, strain MT25^T had a relatively large genome containing genes likely to be involved in the biosynthesis of novel natural products. Bioinformatic analyses of the genome of the *M. provoactoris* strain revealed a broad range of stress-related genes relevant to its survival in deep-sea sediments.

Supplementary Materials: The following are available online at http://www.mdpi.com/xxx/s1, Table S1: 1D and 2D NMR data for compound (1), Figures S1: Photograph of *M. provocatoris* MT25^T and scanning electron micrograph showing single spores, Figure S2: Polar lipid patterns, Figures S3–S11: NMR and mass spectra of compound (1), Table S2: 1D and 2D NMR data for compound (2), Figure S12–S25: NMR and mass spectra of compound (2), Table S3: Some putative stress response genes.

Author Contributions: W.M.A.-M., B.L. and A.V.K. performed whole genome sequencing and bioinformatics analyses. W.M.A.-M., L.H.A.-W. and M.S.M.A.-S. analyzed the sequencing data for protein coding genes and their functions. The acquisition of the phenotypic data on the *M. provocatoris* and the *M. tulbaghiae* strains was carried out by A.B.K. and H.S., A.B.K., H.S., B.L. and A.V.K. performed identification of the strain based on 16S rRNA and whole genome analysis and produced phylogenetic and phylogenomic trees. W.P.-A. isolated and purified the strain from the marine sediment. I.N. and M.G. were responsible for the provision of strain MT25^T and for the isolation and purification of DNA extracted from it. W.M.A.-M. and M.J. cultivated the organism for the isolation and identification of compounds 1 and 2. M.G. and W.P.-A. deposited strain MT25^T in the NCIMB and TISTR culture collections, respectively. W.M.A.-M., L.H.A.-W., B.L., M.S.M.A.-S., M.G., A.B.K., H.S., M.J. and A.V.K. prepared the manuscript. All authors have read and agreed to the published version of the manuscript.

Funding: This work was funded by the Deanship of Scientific Research at Princess Nourah bint Abdulrahman University, through the Research Groups Program Grant no. (RGP-1440-0014) (2).

Institutional Review Board Statement: Not applicable.

Informed Consent Statement: Not applicable.

Data Availability Statement: The article contains all the data produced in this study.

Acknowledgments: This work was funded by the Deanship of Scientific Research at Princess Nourah bint Abdulrahman University, through the Research Groups Program Grant no. (RGP-1440-0014) (2). M.G. is indebted to Jose M. Iqbal (Instituto de Resoursos Naturales Y Agrobilogia de Salamanca, Spain) for undertaking the fatty acid analyses. We thank Anthony Wright for acquiring the NMR data at the Australian Institute of Marine Sciences.

Conflicts of Interest: The authors declare that they do not have any conflict of interest.

References

1. Kamjam, M.; Sivalingam, P.; Deng, Z.; Hong, K. Deep sea actinomycetes and their secondary metabolites. *Front. Microbiol.* **2017**, *8*, 760. [CrossRef] [PubMed]
2. Bull, A.T.; Goodfellow, M. Dark, rare and inspirational microbial matter in the extremobiosphere: 16,000 m of bioprospecting campaigns. *Microbiology* **2019**, *165*, 1252–1264. [CrossRef] [PubMed]
3. Subramani, R.; Sipkema, D. Marine rare actinomycetes: A promising source of structurally diverse and unique novel natural products. *Mar. Drugs* **2019**, *17*, 249. [CrossRef]

4. Riedlinger, J.; Reicke, A.; Zähner, H.; Krismer, B.; Bull, A.T.; Maldonado, L.A.; Ward, A.C.; Goodfellow, M.; Bister, B.; Bischoff, D.; et al. Abyssomicins, inhibitors of the *para*-aminobenzoic acid pathway produced by the marine *Verrucosispora* strain AB-18-032. *J. Antibiot.* **2004**, *57*, 271–279. [CrossRef]
5. Nouioui, I.; Carro, L.; García-López, M.; Meier-Kolthoff, J.P.; Woyke, T.; Kyrpides, N.C.; Pukall, R.; Klenk, H.P.; Goodfellow, M.; Göker, M. Genome-based taxonomic classification of the phylum *Actinobacteria*. *Front. Microbiol.* **2018**, *9*, 2007. [CrossRef]
6. Fiedler, H.P.; Bruntner, C.; Riedlinger, J.; Bull, A.T.; Knutsen, G.; Goodfellow, M.; Jones, A.; Maldonado, L.; Pathom-aree, W.; Beil, W.; et al. Proximicin A, B and C, novel aminofuran antibiotic and anticancer compounds isolated from marine strains of the actinomycete *Verrucosispora*. *J. Antibiot.* **2008**, *61*, 158–163. [CrossRef]
7. Goodfellow, M.; Brown, R.; Ahmed, L.; Pathom-aree, W.; Bull, A.T.; Jones, A.L.; Stach, J.E.; Zucchi, T.D.; Zhang, L.; Wang, J. *Verrucosispora fiedleri* sp. nov., an actinomycete isolated from a fjord sediment which synthesizes proximicins. *Antonie van Leeuwenhoek* **2013**, *103*, 493–502. [CrossRef]
8. Carro, L.; Nouioui, I.; Sangal, V.; Meier-Kolthoff, J.P.; Trujillo, M.E.; Montero-Calasanz, M.D.C.; Sahin, N.; Smith, D.L.; Kim, K.E.; Peluso, P.; et al. Genome-based classification of micromonosporae with a focus on their biotechnological and ecological potential. *Sci. Rep.* **2018**, *8*, 525. [CrossRef]
9. Carro, L.; Castro, J.F.; Razmilic, V.; Nouioui, I.; Pan, C.; Igual, J.M.; Jaspars, M.; Goodfellow, M.; Bull, A.T.; Asenjo, J.A.; et al. Uncovering the potential of novel micromonosporae isolated from an extreme hyper-arid Atacama Desert soil. *Sci. Rep.* **2019**, *9*, 4678. [CrossRef]
10. Carro, L.; Golinska, P.; Nouioui, I.; Bull, A.T.; Igual, J.M.; Andrews, B.A.; Klenk, H.P.; Goodfellow, M. *Micromonospora acroterricola* sp. nov., a novel actinobacterium isolated from a high altitude Atacama Desert soil. *Int. J. Syst. Evol. Microbiol.* **2019**, *69*, 3426–3436. [CrossRef] [PubMed]
11. Tacconelli, E.; Carrara, E.; Savoldi, A.; Harbarth, S.; Mendelson, M.; Monnet, D.L.; Pulcini, C.; Kahlmeter, G.; Kluytmans, J.; Carmeli, Y.; et al. Discovery, research, and development of new antibiotics: The WHO priority list of antibiotic-resistant bacteria and tuberculosis. *Lancet Infect. Dis.* **2018**, *18*, 318–327. [CrossRef]
12. Carro, L.; Razmilic, V.; Nouioui, I.; Richardson, L.; Pan, C.; Golinska, P.; Asenjo, J.A.; Bull, A.T.; Klenk, H.P.; Goodfellow, M. Hunting for cultivable *Micromonospora* strains in soils of the Atacama Desert. *Antonie van Leeuwenhoek* **2018**, *111*, 1375–1387. [CrossRef]
13. Ørskov, J. *Investigations into the Morphology of the Ray Fungi*; Levin and Munksgaard: Copenhagen, Denmark, 1923.
14. Krassilnikov, N.A. *Ray Fungi and Related Organisms, Actinomycetales*; Akademii Nauk S. S. S. R.: Moscow, Russia, 1938.
15. Genilloud, O. Order XI. *Micromonosporales* ord. nov. In *Bergey's Manual of Systematic Bacteriology*, 2nd ed.; Goodfellow, M., Kämpfer, P., Busse, H.-J., Trujillo, M.E., Suzuki, K.-i., Ludwig, W., Whitman, W.B., Eds.; Springer: Berlin/Heidelberg, Germany, 2012; Volume 5, p. 1035.
16. Salam, N.; Jiao, J.Y.; Zhang, X.T.; Li, W.J. Update on the classification of higher ranks in the phylum *Actinobacteria*. *Int. J. Syst. Evol. Microbiol.* **2020**, *70*, 1331–1355. [CrossRef]
17. Foulerton, A.G.R. New species of *Streptothrix* isolated from the air. *Lancet* **1905**, *1*, 1199–1200.
18. Genilloud, O.; Ørskov, G.I.M. 156AL. In *Bergey's Manual of Systematic Bacteriology*, 2nd ed.; Goodfellow, M., Kämpfer, P., Busse, H.-J., Trujillo, M.E., Suzuki, K.-I., Ludwig, W., Whitman, W.B., Eds.; Springer: Berlin/Heidelberg, Germany, 2012; Volume 5, pp. 1039–1057.
19. Pathom-Aree, W.; Stach, J.E.; Ward, A.C.; Horikoshi, K.; Bull, A.T.; Goodfellow, M. Divesity of actinomycetes isolated from Challenger Deep sediment (10,898 m) from the Mariana Trench. *Extremophiles* **2006**, *10*, 181–189. [CrossRef] [PubMed]
20. Vickers, J.C.; Williams, S.T.; Ross, G.W. A taxonomic approach to selective isolation of streptomycetes from soil. In *Biological, Biochemical and Biomedical Aspects of Actinomycetes*; Ortiz-Ortiz, L., Bojalil, L.F., Yakoleff, V., Eds.; Academic Press: Orlando, FL, USA, 1984; pp. 553–561.
21. Kato, C.; Li, L.; Tamaoka, J.; Horikoshi, K. Molecular analyses of the sediment of the 11,000-m deep Mariana Trench. *Extremophiles* **1997**, *1*, 117–123. [CrossRef]
22. Smith, L.T.; Smith, G.M. An osmoregulated dipeptide in stressed *Rhizobium meliloti*. *J. Bacteriol.* **1989**, *171*, 4714–4717. [CrossRef] [PubMed]
23. Masatomi, I.; Tetsuya, S.; Masahide, A.; Ryuichi, S.; Hiroshi, N.; Masaaki, I.; Tomio, T. IC202A, a new siderophore with immunosuppressive activity produced by *Streptoalloteichus* sp. 1454-19. II. Physico-chemical properties and structure elucidation. *J. Antibiot.* **1999**, *52*, 25–28.
24. Tatusova, T.; DiCuccio, M.; Badretdin, A.; Chetvernin, V.; Nawrocki, E.P.; Zaslavsky, L.; Lomsadze, A.; Pruitt, K.D.; Borodovsky, M.; Ostell, J. NCBI prokaryotic genome annotation pipeline. *Nucleic Acids Res.* **2016**, *44*, 6614–6624. [CrossRef]
25. Angiuoli, S.V.; Gussman, A.; Klimke, W.; Cochrane, G.; Field, D.; Garrity, G.; Kodira, C.D.; Kyrpides, N.; Madupu, R.; Markowitz, V.; et al. Toward an online repository of Standard Operating Procedures (SOPs) for (meta) genomic annotation. *OMICS* **2008**, *12*, 137–141. [CrossRef] [PubMed]
26. Tatusova, T.; Ciufo, S.; Fedorov, B.; O'Neill, K.; Tolstoy, I. RefSeq microbial genomes database: New representation and annotation strategy. *Nucleic Acids Res.* **2014**, *42*, D553–D559. [CrossRef] [PubMed]
27. Sveshnikova, M.A.; Maksimova, T.S.; Kudrina, E.S. Species of the genus *Micromonospora* Oerskov, 1923 and their taxonomy. *Mikrobiologiia* **1969**, *38*, 883–893.

28. Tanasupawat, S.; Jongrungruangchok, S.; Kudo, T. *Micromonospora marina* sp. nov., isolated from sea sand. *Int. J. Syst. Evol. Microbiol.* **2010**, *60*, 648–652. [CrossRef] [PubMed]
29. Songsumanus, A.; Tanasupawat, S.; Igarashi, Y.; Kudo, T. *Micromonospora maritima* sp. nov., isolated from mangrove soil. *Int. J. Syst. Evol. Microbiol.* **2013**, *63*, 554–559. [CrossRef]
30. Supong, K.; Suriyachadkun, C.; Tanasupawat, S.; Suwanborirux, K.; Pittayakhajonwut, P.; Kudo, T.; Thawai, C. *Micromonospora sediminicola* sp. nov., isolated from marine sediment. *Int. J. Syst. Evol. Microbiol.* **2013**, *63*, 570–575. [CrossRef] [PubMed]
31. Kirby, B.M.; Meyers, P.R. *Micromonospora tulbaghiae* sp. nov., isolated from the leaves of wild garlic, *Tulbaghia violacea*. *Int. J. Syst. Evol. Microbiol.* **2010**, *60*, 1328–1333. [CrossRef]
32. Contreras-Castro, L.; Maldonado, L.A.; Quintana, E.T.; Carro, L.; Klenk, H.-P. Genomic insight into three marine *Micromonospora* sp. strains from the Gulf of California. *Microbiol. Resour. Announc.* **2019**, *8*, e01673-18. [CrossRef]
33. Riesco, R.; Carro, L.; Román-Ponce, B.; Prieto, C.; Blom, J.; Klenk, H.P.; Normand, P.; Trujillo, M.E. Defining the species *Micromonospora saelicesensis* and *Micromonospora noduli* Under the framework of genomics. *Front. Microbiol.* **2018**, *9*, 1360. [CrossRef]
34. Songsumanus, A.; Tanasupawat, S.; Thawai, C.; Suwanborirux, K.; Kudo, T. *Micromonospora humi* sp. nov., isolated from peat swamp forest soil. *Int. J. Syst. Evol. Microbiol.* **2011**, *61*, 1176–1181. [CrossRef]
35. Richter, M.; Rosselló-Móra, R. Shifting the genomic gold standard for the prokaryotic species definition. *Proc. Natl. Acad. Sci. USA* **2009**, *106*, 19126–19131. [CrossRef]
36. Chun, J.; Oren, A.; Ventosa, A.; Christensen, H.; Arahal, D.R.; da Costa, M.S.; Rooney, A.P.; Yi, H.; Xu, X.W.; De Meyer, S.; et al. Proposed minimal standards for the use of genome data for the taxonomy of prokaryotes. *Int. J. Syst. Evol. Microbiol.* **2018**, *68*, 461–466. [CrossRef]
37. Meier-Kolthoff, J.P.; Auch, A.F.; Klenk, H.P.; Göker, M. Genome sequence-based species delimitation with confidence intervals and improved distance functions. *BMC Bioinform.* **2013**, *14*, 60. [CrossRef] [PubMed]
38. Thompson, D.; Cognat, V.; Goodfellow, M.; Koechler, S.; Heintz, D.; Carapito, C.; Van Dorsselaer, A.; Mahmoud, H.; Sangal, V.; Ismail, W. Phylogenomic classification and biosynthetic potential of the fossil fuel-biodesulfurizing *Rhodococcus* strain IGTS8. *Front. Microbiol.* **2020**, *11*, 1417. [CrossRef]
39. Li, X.; Huang, Y.; Whitman, W.B. The relationship of the whole genome sequence identity to DNA hybridization varies between genera of prokaryotes. *Antonie van Leeuwenhoek* **2015**, *107*, 241–249. [CrossRef]
40. Palmer, M.; Steenkamp, E.T.; Blom, J.; Hedlund, B.P.; Venter, S.N. All ANIs are not created equal: Implications for prokaryotic species boundaries and integration of ANIs into polyphasic taxonomy. *Int. J. Syst. Evol. Microbiol.* **2020**, *70*, 2937–2948. [CrossRef] [PubMed]
41. Meier-Kolthoff, J.P.; Klenk, H.P.; Göker, M. Taxonomic use of DNA G+C content and DNA-DNA hybridization in the genomic age. *Int. J. Syst. Evol. Microbiol.* **2014**, *64*, 352–356. [CrossRef] [PubMed]
42. Blin, K.; Shaw, S.; Steinke, K.; Villebro, R.; Ziemert, N.; Lee, S.Y.; Medema, M.H.; Weber, T. antiSMASH 5.0: Updates to the secondary metabolite genome mining pipeline. *Nucleic Acids Res.* **2019**, *47*, W81–W87.
43. Sosio, M.; Gaspari, E.; Iorio, M.; Pessina, S.; Medema, M.H.; Bernasconi, A.; Simone, M.; Maffioli, S.I.; Ebright, R.H.; Donadio, S. Analysis of the pseudouridimycin biosynthetic pathway provides insights into the formation of c-nucleoside antibiotics. *Cell Chem. Biol.* **2018**, *25*, 540–549.e4. [CrossRef]
44. Wang, X.; Zhou, H.; Chen, H.; Jing, X.; Zheng, W.; Li, R.; Sun, T.; Liu, J.; Fu, J.; Huo, L.; et al. Discovery of recombinases enables genome mining of cryptic biosynthetic gene clusters in *Burkholderiales* species. *Proc. Natl. Acad. Sci. USA* **2018**, *115*, E4255–E4263.
45. Awakawa, T.; Fujita, N.; Hayakawa, M.; Ohnishi, Y.; Horinouchi, S. Characterization of the biosynthesis gene cluster for alkyl-O-dihydrogeranyl-methoxyhydroquinones in *Actinoplanes missouriensis*. *ChemBioChem* **2011**, *12*, 439–448. [CrossRef]
46. Yanai, K.; Murakami, T.; Bibb, M. Amplification of the entire kanamycin biosynthetic gene cluster during empirical strain improvement of *Streptomyces kanamyceticus*. *Proc. Natl. Acad. Sci. USA* **2006**, *103*, 9661–9666. [CrossRef]
47. Shigemori, H.; Komaki, H.; Yazawa, K.; Mikami, Y.; Nemoto, A.; Tanaka, Y.; Sasaki, T.; In, Y.; Ishida, T.; Kobayashi, J.; et al. Brasilicardin A. A novel tricyclic metabolite with potent immunosuppressive activity from actinomycete *Nocardia brasiliensis*. *J. Org. Chem.* **1998**, *63*, 6900–6904. [CrossRef]
48. Ogasawara, Y.; Yackley, B.J.; Greenberg, J.A.; Rogelj, S.; Melançon, C.E., 3rd. Expanding our understanding of sequence-function relationships of type II polyketide biosynthetic gene clusters: Bioinformatics-guided identification of Frankiamicin A from *Frankia* sp. EAN1pec. *PLoS ONE* **2015**, *10*, e0121505. [CrossRef]
49. Abdel-Mageed, W.M.; Juhasz, B.; Lehri, B.; Alqahtani, A.S.; Nouioui, I.; Pech-Puch, D.; Tabudravu, J.N.; Goodfellow, M.; Rodríguez, J.; Jaspars, M.; et al. Whole genome sequence of *Dermacoccus abyssi* MT1.1 isolated from the Challenger Deep of the Mariana Trench reveals phenazine biosynthesis locus and environmental adaptation factors. *Mar. Drugs* **2020**, *18*, 131. [CrossRef] [PubMed]
50. Gumley, A.W.; Inniss, W.E. Cold shock proteins and cold acclimation proteins in the psychrotrophic bacterium *Pseudomonas putida* Q5 and its transconjugant. *Can. J. Microbiol.* **1996**, *42*, 798–803. [CrossRef]
51. Fujii, S.; Nakasone, K.; Horikoshi, K. Cloning of two cold shock genes, cspA and cspG, from the deep-sea psychrophilic bacterium *Shewanella violacea* strain DSS12. *FEMS Microbiol. Lett.* **1999**, *178*, 123–128. [CrossRef] [PubMed]

52. Abdel-Mageed, W.M.; Lehri, B.; Jarmusch, S.A.; Miranda, K.; Al-Wahaibi, L.H.; Stewart, H.A.; Jamieson, A.J.; Jaspars, M.; Karlyshev, A.V. Whole genome sequencing of four bacterial strains from South Shetland Trench revealing biosynthetic and environmental adaptation gene clusters. *Mar. Genom.* **2020**, *54*, 100782. [CrossRef]
53. Lelivelt, M.J.; Kawula, T.H. Hsc66, an Hsp70 homolog in *Escherichia coli*, is induced by cold shock but not by heat shock. *J. Bacteriol.* **1995**, *177*, 4900–4907. [CrossRef]
54. Lee, S.; Sowa, M.E.; Choi, J.M.; Tsai, F.T. The ClpB/Hsp104 molecular chaperone—A protein disaggregating machine. *J. Struct. Biol.* **2004**, *146*, 99–105. [CrossRef] [PubMed]
55. Redder, P.; Hausmann, S.; Khemici, V.; Yasrebi, H.; Linder, P. Bacterial versatility requires DEAD-box RNA helicases. *FEMS Microbiol. Rev.* **2015**, *39*, 392–412. [CrossRef]
56. Chattopadhyay, M.; Jagannadham, M. Maintenance of membrane fluidity in Antarctic bacteria. *Polar Biol.* **2001**, *24*, 386–388.
57. Chattopadhyay, M.K.; Jagannadham, M.V. A branched chain fatty acid promotes cold adaptation in bacteria. *J. Biosci.* **2003**, *28*, 363–364. [CrossRef]
58. Goude, R.; Renaud, S.; Bonnassie, S.; Bernard, T.; Blanco, C. Glutamine, glutamate, and alpha-glucosylglycerate are the major osmotic solutes accumulated by *Erwinia chrysanthemi* strain 3937. *Appl. Environ. Microbiol.* **2004**, *70*, 6535–6541. [CrossRef]
59. Kuhlmann, A.U.; Hoffmann, T.; Bursy, J.; Jebbar, M.; Bremer, E. Ectoine and hydroxyectoine as protectants against osmotic and cold stress: Uptake through the SigB-controlled betaine-choline- carnitine transporter-type carrier EctT from *Virgibacillus pantothenticus*. *J. Bacteriol.* **2011**, *193*, 4699–4708. [CrossRef]
60. Gouffi, K.; Blanco, C. Is the accumulation of osmoprotectant the unique mechanism involved in bacterial osmoprotection? *Int. J. Food Microbiol.* **2000**, *55*, 171–174. [CrossRef]
61. Nau-Wagner, G.; Opper, D.; Rolbetzki, A.; Boch, J.; Kempf, B.; Hoffmann, T.; Bremer, E. Genetic control of osmoadaptive glycine betaine synthesis in *Bacillus subtilis* through the choline-sensing and glycine betaine-responsive GbsR repressor. *J. Bacteriol.* **2012**, *194*, 2703–2714. [CrossRef] [PubMed]
62. Boncompagni, E.; Osteras, M.; Poggi, M.C.; le Rudulier, D. Occurrence of choline and glycine betaine uptake and metabolism in the family *Rhizobiaceae* and their roles in osmoprotection. *Appl. Environ. Microbiol.* **1999**, *65*, 2072–2077. [CrossRef] [PubMed]
63. Sagot, B.; Gaysinski, M.; Mehiri, M.; Guigonis, J.M.; Le Rudulier, D.; Alloing, G. Osmotically induced synthesis of the dipeptide N-acetylglutaminylglutamine amide is mediated by a new pathway conserved among bacteria. *Proc. Natl. Acad. Sci. USA* **2010**, *107*, 12652–12657. [CrossRef] [PubMed]
64. Campanaro, S.; Treu, L.; Valle, G. Protein evolution in deep sea bacteria: An analysis of amino acids substitution rates. *BMC Evol. Biol.* **2008**, *8*, 313. [CrossRef]
65. Goordial, J.; Raymond-Bouchard, I.; Zolotarov, Y.; de Bethencourt, L.; Ronholm, J.; Shapiro, N.; Woyke, T.; Stromvik, M.; Greer, C.; Bakermans, C.; et al. Cold adaptive traits revealed by comparative genomic analysis of the eurypsychrophile *Rhodococcus* sp. JG3 isolated from high elevation McMurdo Dry Valley permafrost, Antarctica. *FEMS Microbiol. Ecol.* **2016**, *92*, fiv154.
66. Bartlett, D.H. Microbial adaptations to the psychrosphere/piezosphere. *J. Mol. Microbiol. Biotechnol.* **1999**, *1*, 93–100.
67. Sekar, K.; Linker, S.M.; Nguyen, J.; Grünhagen, A.; Stocker, R.; Sauer, U. Bacterial glycogen provides short-term benefits in changing environments. *Appl. Environ. Microbiol.* **2020**, *86*, e00049-20. [CrossRef]
68. Cannon, G.C.; Heinhorst, S.; Kerfeld, C.A. Carboxysomal carbonic anhydrases: Structure and role in microbial CO_2 fixation. *Biochim. Biophys. Acta* **2010**, *1804*, 382–392. [CrossRef]
69. Busarakam, K.; Bull, A.T.; Trujillo, M.E.; Riesco, R.; Sangal, V.; van Wezel, G.P.; Goodfellow, M. *Modestobacter caceresii* sp. nov., novel actinobacteria with an insight into their adaptive mechanisms for survival in extreme hyper-arid Atacama Desert soils. *Syst. Appl. Microbiol.* **2016**, *39*, 243–251. [CrossRef]
70. Castro, J.F.; Nouioui, I.; Sangal, V.; Choi, S.; Yang, S.J.; Kim, B.Y.; Trujillo, M.E.; Riesco, R.; Montero-Calasanz, M.D.C.; Rahmani, T.P.D.; et al. *Blastococcus atacamensis* sp. nov., a novel strain adapted to life in the Yungay core region of the Atacama Desert. *Int. J. Syst. Evol. Microbiol.* **2018**, *68*, 2712–2721. [CrossRef] [PubMed]
71. Castro, J.F.; Nouioui, I.; Sangal, V.; Trujillo, M.E.; Montero-Calasanz, M.D.C.; Rahmani, T.; Bull, A.T.; Asenjo, J.A.; Andrews, B.A.; Goodfellow, M. *Geodermatophilus chilensis* sp. nov., from soil of the Yungay core-region of the Atacama Desert, Chile. *Syst. Appl. Microbiol.* **2018**, *41*, 427–436. [CrossRef] [PubMed]
72. Golińska, P.; Świecimska, M.; Montero-Calasanz, M.D.C.; Yaramis, A.; Igual, J.M.; Bull, A.T.; Goodfellow, M. *Modestobacter altitudinis* sp. nov., a novel actinobacterium isolated from Atacama Desert soil. *Int. J. Syst. Evol. Microbiol.* **2020**, *70*, 3513–3527. [CrossRef]
73. Golinska, P.; Montero-Calasanz, M.D.C.; Świecimska, M.; Yaramis, A.; Igual, J.M.; Bull, A.T.; Goodfellow, M. *Modestobacter excelsi* sp. nov., a novel actinobacterium isolated from a high altitude Atacama Desert soil. *Syst. Appl. Microbiol.* **2020**, *43*, 126051. [CrossRef] [PubMed]
74. Goodfellow, M.; Williams, S.T. Ecology of actinomycetes. *Annu. Rev. Microbiol.* **1983**, *37*, 189–216. [CrossRef] [PubMed]
75. Zenova, G.M.; Zviagintsev, D.G. Aktinomitsety roda *Micromonospora* v lugovykh ékosistemakh [Actinomycetes of the genus *Micromonospora* in meadow ecosystems]. *Mikrobiologiia* **2002**, *71*, 662–666.
76. Hong, K.; Gao, A.H.; Xie, Q.Y.; Gao, H.; Zhuang, L.; Lin, H.P.; Yu, H.P.; Li, J.; Yao, X.S.; Goodfellow, M.; et al. Actinomycetes for marine drug discovery isolated from mangrove soils and plants in China. *Mar. Drugs* **2009**, *7*, 24–44. [CrossRef] [PubMed]
77. Lee, I.; Chalita, M.; Ha, S.M.; Na, S.I.; Yoon, S.H.; Chun, J. ContEst16S: An algorithm that identifies contaminated prokaryotic genomes using 16S RNA gene sequences. *Int. J. Syst. Evol. Microbiol.* **2017**, *67*, 2053–2057. [CrossRef] [PubMed]

78. Yoon, S.H.; Ha, S.M.; Kwon, S.; Lim, J.; Kim, Y.; Seo, H.; Chun, J. Introducing EzBioCloud: A taxonomically united database of 16S rRNA gene sequences and whole-genome assemblies. *Int. J. Syst. Evol. Microbiol.* **2017**, *67*, 1613–1617. [CrossRef] [PubMed]
79. Edgar, R.C. MUSCLE: Multiple sequence alignment with high accuracy and high throughput. *Nucleic Acids Res.* **2004**, *32*, 1792–1797. [CrossRef] [PubMed]
80. Meier-Kolthoff, J.P.; Göker, M.; Spröer, C.; Klenk, H.P. When should a DDH experiment be mandatory in microbial taxonomy? *Arch. Microbiol.* **2013**, *195*, 413–418. [CrossRef]
81. Felsenstein, J. Evolutionary trees from DNA sequences: A maximum likelihood approach. *J. Mol. Evol.* **1981**, *17*, 368–376. [CrossRef]
82. Fitch, W. Toward defining the course of evolution: Minimum change for a specific tree topology. *Syst. Zool.* **1971**, *20*, 406–416. [CrossRef]
83. Saitou, N.; Nei, M. The neighbor-joining method: A new method for reconstructing phylogenetic trees. *Mol. Biol. Evol.* **1987**, *4*, 406–425.
84. Stamatakis, A. RAxML version 8: A tool for phylogenetic analysis and post-analysis of large phylogenies. *Bioinformatics* **2014**, *30*, 1312–1313. [CrossRef]
85. Pattengale, N.D.; Alipour, M.; Bininda-Emonds, O.R.; Moret, B.M.; Stamatakis, A. How many bootstrap replicates are necessary? *J. Comput. Biol.* **2010**, *17*, 337–354. [CrossRef]
86. Goloboff, P.A.; Farris, J.S.; Nixon, K.C. TNT, a free program for phylogenetic analysis. *Cladistics* **2008**, *24*, 774–786. [CrossRef]
87. Swofford, D.L. *PAUP*. *Phylogenetic analysis using parsimony (*and Other Methods)*; Vers. 4; Sinauer: Sunderland, MA, USA, 1998.
88. Felsenstein, J. Confidence limits on phylogenies: An approach using the bootstrap. *Evolution* **1985**, *39*, 783–791. [CrossRef] [PubMed]
89. Kumar, S.; Stecher, G.; Li, M.; Knyaz, C.; Tamura, K. MEGA X: Molecular evolutionary genetics analysis across computing platforms. *Mol. Biol. Evol.* **2018**, *35*, 1547–1549. [CrossRef]
90. Jukes, T.; Cantor, C. Evolution of protein molecules. In *Mammalian Protein Metabolism*; Volume III. Chapter 24; Munro, H., Ed.; Academic Press: New York, NY, USA, 1969; pp. 21–132.
91. Staneck, J.L.; Roberts, G.D. Simplified approach to identification of aerobic actinomycetes by thin-layer chromatography. *Appl. Microbiol.* **1974**, *28*, 226–231. [CrossRef] [PubMed]
92. Lechevalier, M.P.; Lechevalier, H. Chemical composition as a criterion in the classification of aerobic actinomycetes. *Int. J. Syst. Bacteriol.* **1970**, *20*, 435–443. [CrossRef]
93. Minnikin, D.E.; O'Donnell, A.G.; Goodfellow, M.; Alderson, G.; Athalye, M.; Schaal, A.; Parlett, J.H. An integrated procedure for the extraction of bacterial isoprenoid quinones and polar lipids. *J. Microbiol. Methods* **1984**, *2*, 233–241. [CrossRef]
94. Kroppenstedt, B.M.; Goodfellow, M. The family *Thermomonosporaceae*, *Actinocorallia*, *Spirillospora* and *Thermomonospora*. In *The Prokaryotes*, 2nd ed.; Volume 3: Archaea. Bacteria: Firmicutes, Actinomycetes; Dworkin, M., Falkow, S., Schleifer, K.-H., Stackebrandt, E., Eds.; Springer: Berlin/Heidelberg, Germany, 2006; pp. 682–724.
95. Shirling, E.B.; Gottlieb, D. Methods for characterization of *Streptomyces* species. *Int. J. Syst. Bacteriol.* **1966**, *16*, 313–340. [CrossRef]
96. Sasser, M. *Identification of Bacteria by Gas Chromatography of Cellular Fatty Acids*; MIDI Technical Note; MIDI: Newark, DE, USA, 1990; Volume 101, p. 1.
97. O'Donnell, A.G.; Falconer, C.; Goodfellow, M.; Ward, A.C.; Williams, E. Biosystematics and diversity amongst novel carboxydotrophic actinomycetes. *Antonie van Leeuwenhoek* **1993**, *64*, 325–340. [CrossRef]
98. Williams, S.T.; Goodfellow, M.; Alderson, G.; Wellington, E.M.H.; Sneath, P.H.A.; Sackin, M.J. Numerical classification of *Streptomyces* and related genera. *J. Gen. Microbiol.* **1983**, *129*, 1743–1813. [CrossRef]
99. Lehmann, P.F.; Murray, P.R.; Baron, E.J.; Pfaller, M.A.; Tenover, F.C.; Yolken, R.H. (Eds.) *Manual of Clinical Microbiology*, 7th ed.; Sigma-Aldrich: St. Louis, MO, USA, 2015; Volume 146, pp. 107–108. [CrossRef]
100. Ausubel, F.M.; Brent, R.; Kingston, R.E.; Moore, D.D.; Seidman, J.G.; Smith, J.A.; Struhl, K. *Current Protocols in Molecular Biology*; John Wiley and Sons, Inc.: New York, NY, USA, 1994.
101. Altschul, S.F.; Gish, W.; Miller, W.; Myers, E.W.; Lipman, D.J. Basic local alignment search tool. *J. Mol. Biol.* **1990**, *215*, 403–410. [CrossRef]
102. Wattam, A.R.; Davis, J.J.; Assaf, R.; Boisvert, S.; Brettin, T.; Bun, C.; Conrad, N.; Dietrich, E.M.; Disz, T.; Gabbard, J.L.; et al. Improvements to PATRIC, the all-bacterial Bioinformatics Database and Analysis Resource Center. *Nucleic Acids Res.* **2017**, *45*, D535–D542. [CrossRef] [PubMed]
103. Lee, I.; Ouk Kim, Y.; Park, S.C.; Chun, J. OrthoANI: An improved algorithm and software for calculating average nucleotide identity. *Int. J. Syst. Evol. Microbiol.* **2016**, *66*, 1100–1103. [CrossRef] [PubMed]

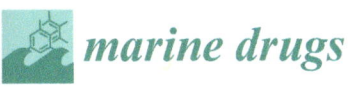

Article

New from Old: Thorectandrin Alkaloids in a Southern Australian Marine Sponge, *Thorectandra choanoides* (CMB-01889)

Shamsunnahar Khushi, Angela A. Salim, Ahmed H. Elbanna, Laizuman Nahar and Robert J. Capon *

Institute for Molecular Bioscience, The University of Queensland, St. Lucia, QLD 4072, Australia; s.khushi@imb.uq.edu.au (S.K.); a.salim@uq.edu.au (A.A.S.); a.elbanna@imb.uq.edu.au (A.H.E.); laboni4@yahoo.com (L.N.)
* Correspondence: r.capon@uq.edu.au; Tel.: +61-7-3346-2979

Citation: Khushi, S.; Salim, A.A.; Elbanna, A.H.; Nahar, L.; Capon, R.J. New from Old: Thorectandrin Alkaloids in a Southern Australian Marine Sponge, *Thorectandra choanoides* (CMB-01889). *Mar. Drugs* **2021**, *19*, 97. https://doi.org/10.3390/md19020097

Academic Editor: Kazuo Umezawa

Received: 10 January 2021
Accepted: 5 February 2021
Published: 9 February 2021

Publisher's Note: MDPI stays neutral with regard to jurisdictional claims in published maps and institutional affiliations.

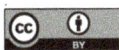

Copyright: © 2021 by the authors. Licensee MDPI, Basel, Switzerland. This article is an open access article distributed under the terms and conditions of the Creative Commons Attribution (CC BY) license (https://creativecommons.org/licenses/by/4.0/).

Abstract: *Thorectandra choanoides* (CMB-01889) was prioritized as a source of promising new chemistry from a library of 960 southern Australian marine sponge extracts, using a global natural products social (GNPS) molecular networking approach. The sponge was collected at a depth of 45 m. Chemical fractionation followed by detailed spectroscopic analysis led to the discovery of a new tryptophan-derived alkaloid, thorectandrin A (**1**), with the GNPS cluster revealing a halo of related alkaloids **1a–1n**. In considering biosynthetic origins, we propose that *Thorectandra choanoides* (CMB-01889) produces four well-known alkaloids, 6-bromo-1′,8-dihydroaplysinopsin (**2**), 6-bromoaplysinopsin (**3**), aplysinopsin (**4**), and 1′,8-dihydroaplysinopsin (**10**), all of which are susceptible to processing by a putative indoleamine 2,3-dioxygenase-*like* (IDO) enzyme to **1a–1n**. Where the 1′,8-dihydroalkaloids **2** and **10** are fully transformed to stable ring-opened thorectandrins **1** and **1a–1b**, and **1h–1j**, respectively, the conjugated precursors **3** and **4** are transformed to highly reactive Michael acceptors that during extraction and handling undergo complete transformation to artifacts **1c–1g**, and **1k–1n**, respectively. Knowledge of the susceptibility of aplysinopsins as substrates for IDOs, and the relative reactivity of Michael acceptor transformation products, informs our understanding of the pharmaceutical potential of this vintage marine pharmacophore. For example, the cancer tissue specificity of IDOs could be exploited for an immunotherapeutic response, with aplysinopsins transforming in situ to Michael acceptor thorectandrins, which covalently bind and inhibit the enzyme.

Keywords: *Thorectandra choanoides*; tryptophan alkaloid; indoleamine 2,3-dioxygenase; aplysinopsins; GNPS molecular network

1. Introduction

Marine sponges of the genus *Thorectandra* are a rich source of structurally diverse metabolites with novel scaffolds. Examples include, the 1988 report of the sesterterpenes manoalide 25-monoacetate and thorectolide 25-monoacetate from *Thorectandra excavates* collected near Darwin, Australia [1]; the 1995 report of a furanoditerpene from a Southern Australian *Thorectandra choanoides* [2]; and the 2001 and 2002 reports of sesterterpenes thorectandoles A–E from a Palauan *Thorectandra* sp. [3,4]. In addition to terpenes, many alkaloids were also reported from *Thorectandra* sp., including β-carboline alkaloids (i.e., thorectandramine [5], 1-deoxysecofascaplysin A, and fascaplysin [6]), tryptophan alkaloids (i.e., 1′,8-dihydroaplysinopsin and (1*H*-indole-3-yl)acetic acid [7]), and brominated tryptophan alkaloids (i.e., 6-bromo-1′,8-dihydroaplysinopsin, 6-bromo-1′-hydroxy-1′,8-dihydro-aplysinopsin, 6-bromo-1′-methoxy-1′,8-dihydroaplysinopsin, (−)-5-bromo-*N,N*-dimethyl-tryptophan, and (+)-5-bromohypaphorine [7]).

Recently, a GNPS molecular networking analysis was employed on 960 Southern Australian marine sponges, to map the chemical space of natural products, which resulted in the isolation of rare indolo-imidazole alkaloids, trachycladindoles H–M [8], new sesterterpene butenolides, cacolides A–L and cacolic acids A–C [9], and new sesquiterpenes, dysidealactams A–F, and dysidealactones A–B [10]. In this report, we present the discovery of a new class of tryptophan-derived alkaloid, thorectandrin A (**1**) (Figure 1), from a Great Australian Bight specimen of *Thorectandra choanoides*, prioritized for chemical investigation, based on GNPS molecular networking analysis of the same library of Southern Australian sponges.

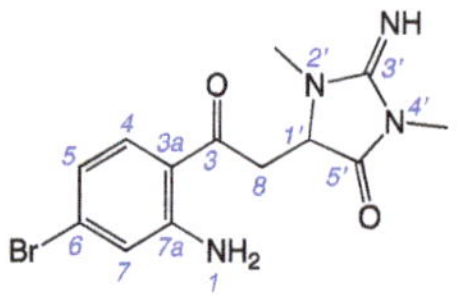

Figure 1. Thorectandrin A (**1**).

2. Results and Discussion

2.1. GNPS Molecular Networking to Explore New Chemistry

To search for new marine natural products, 960 *n*-BuOH soluble partitions from the EtOH extracts of a library of Southern Australian marine sponges and 95 authentic standards (previously isolated from marine sponges) from the Capon lab were assembled and subjected to UPLC-QTOF-MS/MS analysis. The resulting data were used to create a consolidated GNPS molecular network (Figure S1). In this molecular network, we found a specific molecular cluster (Figure S2) associated with *Thorectandra choanoides* (CMB-01889) (collected in 1995 during deep water scientific trawling in the Great Australian Bight), which did not co-correlate with any metabolites found in the other 959 sponge extracts, or any of our authentic marine natural products. Following isolation, detailed spectroscopic analysis identified a new alkaloid scaffold, thorectandrin A (**1**) (Figure 1), while mass spectrometry (MS) data revealed molecular formulae for a host of structurally related analogues (**1a–1n**) in the same GNPS cluster. Note: All *Thorectandra choanoides* (CMB-01889) chemistry in this report are displayed as free bases, although all were isolated, and where appropriate, characterised as the trifluoroacetic acid salts.

2.2. Thorectandrin A (**1**)

HRESI (+) MS analysis of **1** returned a molecular formula ($C_{13}H_{15}BrN_4O_2$, Δmmu +2.6) incorporating eight double-bond equivalents (DBE). The NMR (methanol-d_4) data for **1** (Table 1, Figures S5–S10) revealed resonances attributed to a ketone (δ_C 197.8, C-3), two sp^2 amido/imino carbonyl carbons (δ_C 160.3, C-3′ and 173.8, C-5′), and a 1,2,4-trisubstituted aromatic ring (δ_C 154.1, C-7a; 133.9, C-4, 131.1, C-6; 120.7, C-7; 119.4, C-5; 116.1, C-3a; δ_H 7.67, d, J = 8.7 Hz, H-4; 6.73, br d, J = 8.7 Hz, H-5 and 6.97, br s, H-7), accounting for seven DBE, and requiring that **1** incorporate an additional ring system. Further analysis of NMR data revealed resonances for two *N*-methyls (δ_H 3.09, s, 2′*N*-Me and 3.26, s, 4′*N*-Me) and a deshielded diastereotopic methylene-methine spin system (δ_H 3.94, dd, J = 19.0 and 3.5 Hz, H-8a; 3.67, dd, J = 19.0 and 3.9 Hz, H-8b; and 4.56, dd, J = 3.9 and 3.5 Hz, H-1′). HMBC correlations from 2′*N*-Me and 4′*N*-Me to a common C-3′ guanidino carbon; from 4′*N*-Me and H-1′ to a common carbonyl C-5′ and from 2′*N*-Me to C-1′ (δ_C 60.8) suggested the presence of a 2-imino-1,3-dimethylimidazolidin-4-one ring system, similar to that observed in the well-known *Thorectandra* metabolite aplysinopsin [11]. HMBC correlations from H-4, H-8a, H-8b, and H-1′ to C-3 confirmed that the aromatic ring was connected to the imidazolidinone ring, through a common carbon C-3, establishing the structure of thorectandrin A (**1**), as shown (Figure 2). Comparison of 1D and 2D NMR data of **1** with that of the known sponge metabolite 6-bromo-1′,8-dihydroaplysinopsin (**2**) [7] (Figure 2) revealed the main differences as the disappearance of resonances for H-2/C-2 (δ_H 7.09, δ_C 124.8) in **2** and replacement of the resonance of an sp^2 carbon C-3 (δ_C 106.5) in **2** with an α,β-unsaturated ketone (δ_C 197.8) in **1**, consistent with a ring-opened analogue of **2**.

Table 1. NMR (600 MHz) data for thorectandrin A (1) in methanol-d_4.

Position	δ_C	δ_H, Mult. (J in Hz)	COSY	HMBC	ROESY
3	197.8				
3a	116.1				
4	133.9	7.67, d (8.7)	5	6, 7a, 3	8a, 8b
5	119.4	6.73, br d (8.7)	4,7	3a, 7	
6	131.1				
7	120.7	6.97, br s	5	3a, 5, 6	
7a	154.1				
8	38.0	a. 3.94, dd (19.0, 3.5)	8b, 1'	1', 5', 3	4
		b. 3.67, dd (19.0, 3.9)	8a, 1'	1', 3	4
1'	60.8	4.56, dd (3.9, 3.5)	8a, 8b	5', 3	2'N-CH$_3$
2'N-CH$_3$	30.3	3.09, s		3', 1'	1'
3'	160.3				
4'N-CH$_3$	26.8	3.26, s		3', 5'	
5'	173.8				

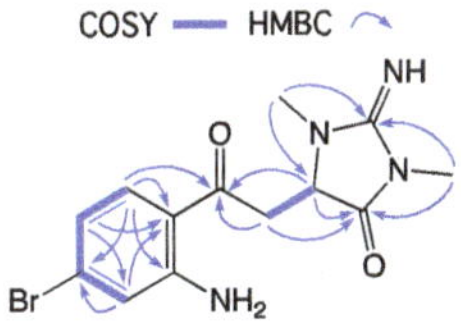

Figure 2. Diagnostic 2D NMR correlations for thorectandrin A (1).

As thorectandrin A (1) did not exhibit a measurable $[\alpha]_D$ or ECD spectrum (Figure S12), we propose it exists as a racemate, induced by a slow keto-enol tautomerization during long-term storage (~25 years) in EtOH (Scheme 1). That the proposed racemization is slow was evident when 1 did not incorporate deuterium, when stored in deuterated methanol for several days.

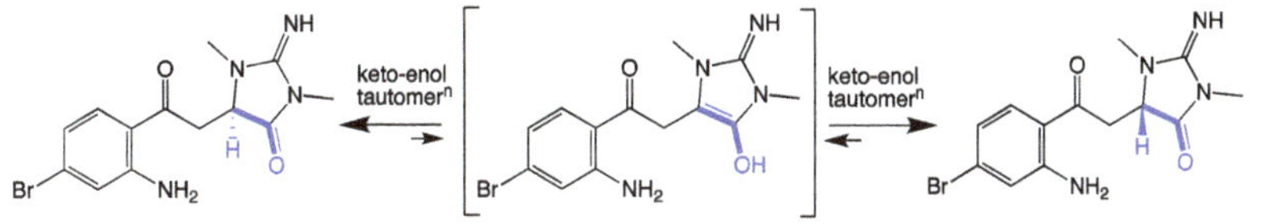

Scheme 1. Keto-enol tautomerization of thorectandrin A (1).

Thorectandrin A (1) did not exhibit growth inhibitory activity against the Gram-positive bacterium *Bacillus subtilis* (ATCC 6051), the Gram-negative *Escherichia coli* (ATCC 11775), the fungus *Candida albicans* (ATCC 10231), or human colorectal (SW620) and lung (NCI-H460) carcinoma cells, at concentrations up to 30 µM (Figures S13 and S14).

2.3. Plausible Biosynthetic Pathway

Aplysinopsins are tryptophan-derived marine natural products, which were isolated from many genera of sponges and scleractinian corals, as well as from one sea anemone and one nudibranch [11], the latter most likely a dietary input from nudibranches feeding on sponges. Typical exemplars include 6-bromoaplysinopsin (3) and aplysinopsin (4). In turning our attention to the likely biosynthesis of thorectandrin A (1), we considered the metabolic relationship between L-tryptophan (5), N-formyl-L-kynurenine (6), and L-kynurenine (7), and the fact that indoleamine 2,3-dioxygenase is known to convert 5 to 6, which undergoes facile hydrolysis by a formamidase to 7 (Scheme 2) [12].

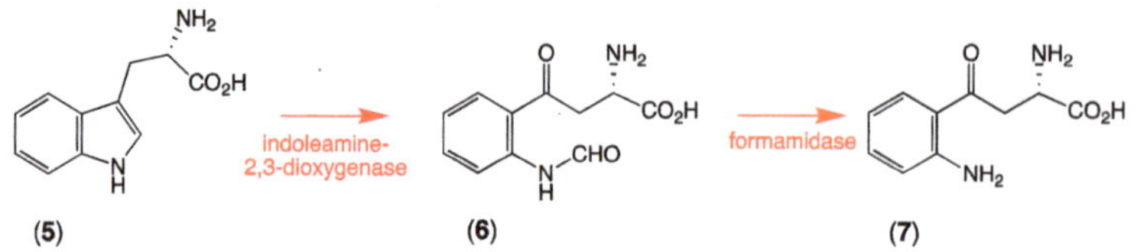

Scheme 2. Biosynthetic conversion of L-tryptophan (**5**) to *N*-formyl-L-kynurenine (**6**) to L-kynurenine (**7**).

Inspired by this sequence of transformations, we hypothesised that a comparable indoleamine 2,3-dioxygenase-*like* enzyme in *Thorectandra choanoides* (CMB-01889) converts 6-bromo-1′,8-dihydroaplysinopsin (**2**) to its ring-opened *N*-formyl derivative (**1a**), which is then rapidly hydrolyzed to thorectandrin A (**1**) (Scheme 3). Although **2** is reported as a sponge natural product [7], its absolute configuration (even enantiopurity) remains unassigned. Based on our experience, a possible challenge to assigning an absolute configuration to **2** might be enantiopurity, due to a propensity for keto-enol mediated epimerisation/racemisation.

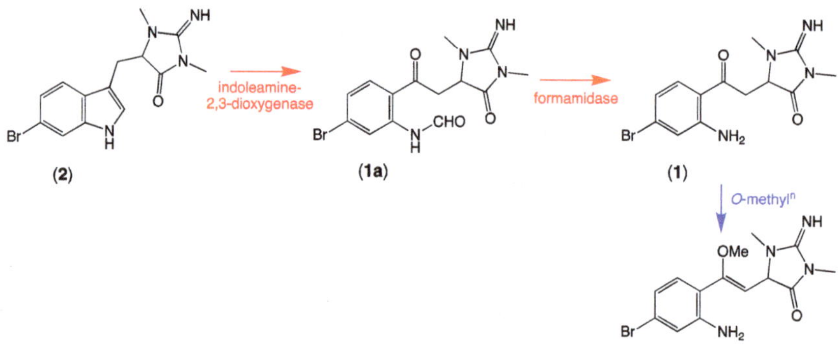

Scheme 3. Possible biosynthetic link between 6-bromo-1′,8-dihydroaplysinopsin (**2**), *N*-formyl thorectandrin A (**1a**), *O*-methylthorectandrin A (**1b**), and thorectandrin A (**1**).

Armed with knowledge of the new thorectandrin scaffold and its likely biosynthetic relationship to the vintage aplysinopsin scaffold, we turned our attention to the literature and noted a 2015 report of racemic spiroreticulatine (**8**) from the South China Sea marine sponge *Fascaplysinopsis reticulata* [13], and a subsequent 2019 report from the same source of the known sponge alkaloid (*Z*)-3′-deimino-3′-oxoaplysinopsin (**9**), as a co-metabolite with **1b** [14]. Although **8** was initially ascribed a plausible biosynthesis involving condensation of indole-3-carboxaldehyde and 1,3-dimethylhydantoin, this hypothesis seems highly improbable. A far more likely pathway would see ring opening of the indole heterocycle in the cometabolite **9**, delivering a reactive Michael acceptor intermediate that undergoes non-stereoselective (enzyme or non-enzyme mediated) intramolecular Michael addition to racemic **8** (see Scheme 4).

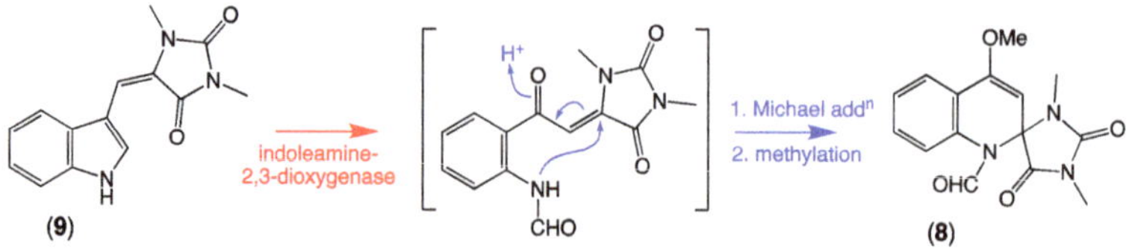

Scheme 4. Possible biosynthetic link between (*Z*)-3′-deimino-3′-oxoaplysinopsin (**9**) and spiroreticulatine (**8**).

2.4. Other Thorectandrin Co-Metabolites

While the thorectandrin GNPS cluster revealed a number of related metabolites, due to low abundance and a lack of sponge biomass, it was not possible to isolate and acquire definitive spectroscopic data to secure unambiguous structure assignments. Notwithstanding, we did acquire molecular formulae for many minor compounds, and on the basis of these measurements and biosynthetic considerations we tentatively propose structures, as shown in Table 2 and Figure 3. For example, based on differences in MW and elemental composition with **1**, we detected a node attributed to the hypothesized N-formyl **1a** (M + H m/z 367, $C_{14}H_{15}BrN_4O_3$) and O-methyl **1b** (M + H m/z 353, $C_{14}H_{17}BrN_4O_2$) (Scheme 3).

Table 2. Molecular formulae of compounds within the thorectandrin GNPS cluster.

m/z [a] (M + H)	Molecular Formula	ΔmDa [b]	MF Difference with 1
	Bromo natural products		
339 (**1**)	$C_{13}H_{15}BrN_4O_2$	0.05	
367 (**1a**)	$C_{14}H_{15}BrN_4O_3$	−1.99	CO
353 (**1b**)	$C_{14}H_{17}BrN_4O_2$	0.78	CH_2
	Bromo natural product solvolysis adducts		
397 (**1c**)	$C_{15}H_{17}BrN_4O_4$	−1.64	$CO + CH_2O$
355 (**1d**)	$C_{13}H_{15}BrN_4O_3$	0.29	O
369 (**1e**)	$C_{14}H_{17}BrN_4O_3$	−1.03	CH_2O
383 (**1f**)	$C_{15}H_{19}BrN_4O_3$	−0.04	C_2H_4O
411 (**1g**)	$C_{17}H_{23}BrN_4O_3$	−0.50	C_4H_8O
	Debromo natural products		
289 (**1h**)	$C_{14}H_{16}N_4O_3$	0.71	−Br + H + CO
261 (**1i**)	$C_{13}H_{16}N_4O_2$	−0.57	−Br + H
303 (**1j**)	$C_{15}H_{18}N_4O_3$	1.2	$−Br + H + CH_2$
	Debromo natural product solvolysis adducts		
277 (**1k**)	$C_{13}H_{16}N_4O_3$	−1.25	−Br + H + O
319 (**1m**)	$C_{15}H_{18}N_4O_4$	1.1	$−Br + H + CO + OCH_2$

[a] m/z from GNPS nodes; [b] Difference between calculated and experimental m/z the latter measured individually from UPLC-QTOF data; NOTE: **1l** (M + H, m/z 305) and **1n** (M + H, m/z 321) are minor metabolites that precluded unambiguous measurement of accurate m/z and MF.

We also detected nodes that were *tentatively* attributed to a methanol (**1c**, M + H m/z 397, $C_{15}H_{17}BrN_4O_4$) adduct of **1a**, and water (**1d**, M + H m/z 355, $C_{13}H_{15}BrN_4O_3$), methanol (**1e**, M + H m/z 369, $C_{14}H_{17}BrN_4O_3$), ethanol (**1f**, M + H m/z 383, $C_{15}H_{19}BrN_4O_3$), and n-butanol (**1g**, M + H m/z 411, $C_{17}H_{23}BrN_4O_3$) adducts of **1** (Table 2, Figure 3). While these adducts **1c–1g** are believed to be solvolysis artifacts induced by long-term storage of *Thorectandra choanoides* (CMB-01889) in aqueous ethanol, followed by n-butanol partitioning and the use of methanol to dissolve dried extract, the absence of a rational solvolysis pathway from **1a** to **1c**, and **1** to **1d–1g**, warranted consideration. We hypothesized that in addition to 6-bromo-1′,8-dihydroaplysinopsin (**2**), *Thorectandra choanoides* (CMB-01889) produces 6-bromoaplysinopsin (**3**), which was comparably transformed by an indoleamine 2,3-dioxygenase-*like* enzyme to reactive Michael adducts (N-formyl-$\Delta^{1'-8}$-thorectandrin A and $\Delta^{1'-8}$-thorectandrin A), with both undergoing Michael addition solvolysis during storage, fractionation and handling, to **1c–1g** (Scheme 5). A recent review highlights the prevalence of solvolysis adduct artifacts among marine natural products, including among imidazoles/imidazolones [15].

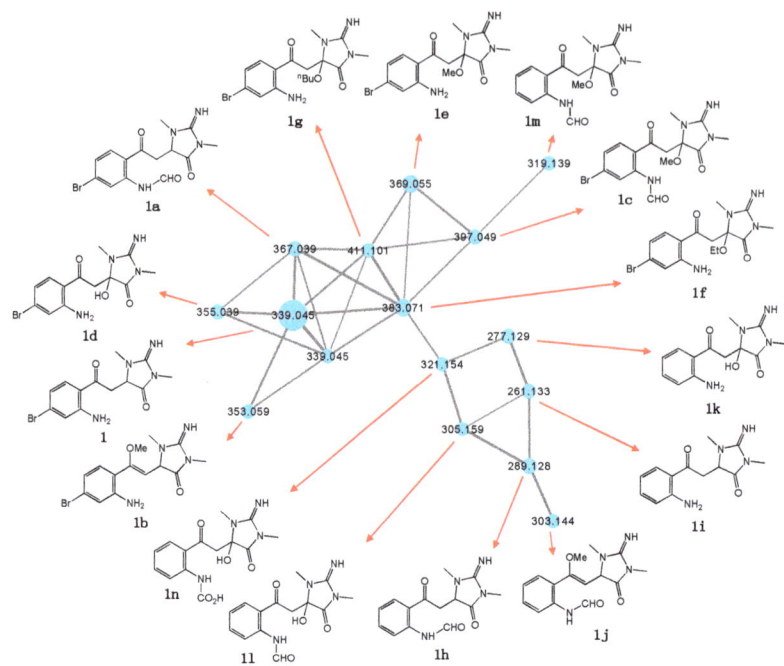

Figure 3. Structures attributed to nodes in the thorectandrin GNPS cluster.

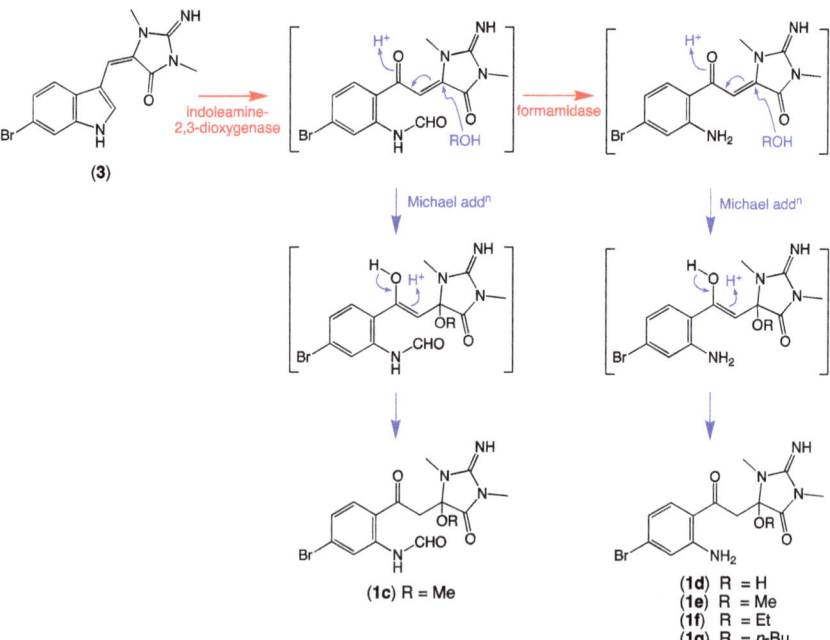

Scheme 5. Possible biosynthetic link between 6-bromoaplysinopsin (**3**) and the solvolysis artifacts **1c–1g**.

Of note, the thorectandrin GNPS cluster also featured nodes tentatively attributed to debromo analogues (**1h**, M + H m/z 289, $C_{14}H_{16}N_4O_3$; **1i**, M + H m/z 261, $C_{13}H_{16}N_4O_2$) **1j**, M + H m/z 303, $C_{15}H_{18}N_4O_3$), consistent with indoleamine 2,3-dioxygenase-like enzyme transformation of 1′,8-dihydroaplysinopsin (**10**) (Scheme 6, Table 2, Figure 3). It also revealed nodes tentatively attributed to solvolysis adduct (**1k**, M + H m/z 277, $C_{13}H_{16}N_4O_3$; **1l**, M + H m/z 305; **1m**, M + H m/z 319, $C_{15}H_{18}N_4O_5$; **1n**, M + H m/z 321), derived from intermediates generated by indoleamine 2,3-dioxygenase-like transformation of aplysinopsin (**4**) (Scheme 7, Table 2, Figure 3).

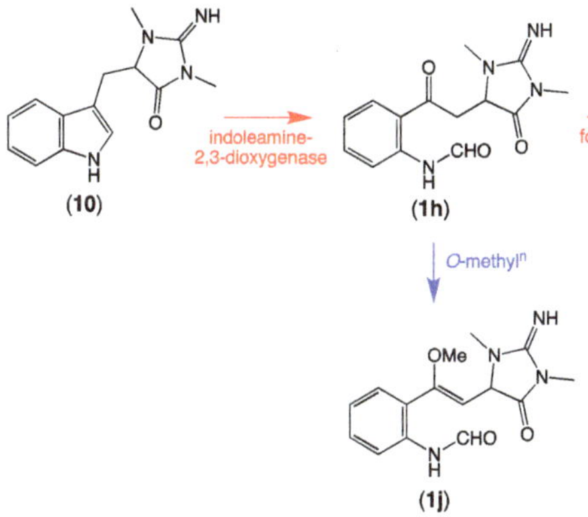

Scheme 6. Possible biosynthetic link between 1′,8-dihydroaplysinopsin (**10**) and **1h–1j**.

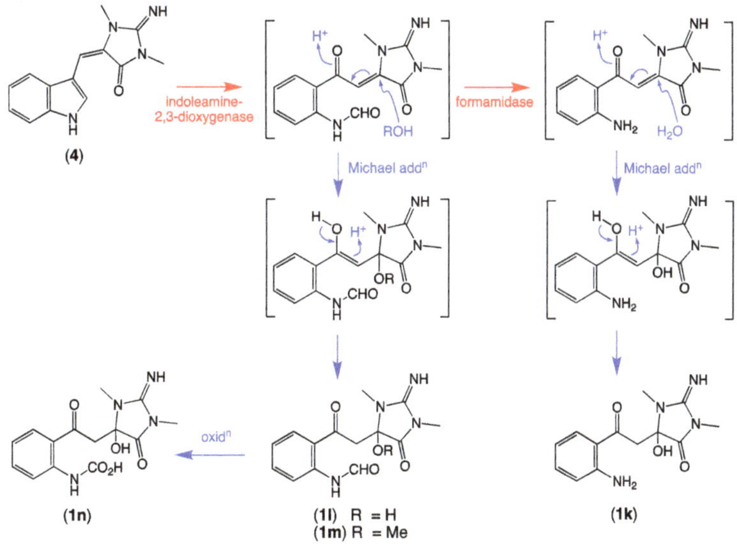

Scheme 7. Possible biosynthetic link between aplysinopsin (**4**) and **1k–1n**.

3. Conclusions

Our application of the GNPS molecular networking to a library of Southern Australian marine sponges reinforced the value of this approach, in both dereplicating and prioritizing extracts for detailed investigation, and in guiding the discovery of new scaffolds. It also revealed itself to be a valuable tool for interrogating the halo of co-clustering minor analogues (including solvolysis artifacts), chemistry that typically defines traditional methods of isolation and structure elucidation.

Our study of an Australian deep water (45 m) marine sponge, *Thorectandra choanoides* (CMB-01889), lead to the discovery of a new class of alkaloid, thorectandrin A (**1**). In proposing a biosynthetic origin of **1**, we speculated that *Thorectandra choanoides* (CMB-01889) possesses enzymes functionally related to indoleamine 2,3-dioxygenase, leading to transformation of the known (albeit rare and minor) sponge natural product 6-bromo-1',8-dihydroaplysinopsin (**2**) to its ring-opened *N*-formyl derivative **1a**, which was then rapidly hydrolyzed to thorectandrin A (**1**). Supportive of this hypothesis, we tentatively identified **1a** in the thorectandrin GNPS cluster, along with the *O*-methyl product **1b**, debromo analogues **1h–1j**, solvolysis adducts **1c–1g** and **1k–1m**, and a natural/artifact oxidation product **1n**. Studies into minor solvolysis artifacts led us to speculate that *Thorectandra choanoides* (CMB-01889) was capable of producing four known alkaloids, 6-bromo-1',8-dihydroaplysinopsin (**2**) [7], 6-bromoaplysinopsin (**3**) [7], aplysinopsin (**4**) [16], and 1',8-dihydroaplysinopsin (**10**) [7], all of which were susceptible to a sponge indoleamine 2,3-dioxygenase-like enzyme. Where the 1',8-dihydro alkaloids **2** and **10** were fully transformed by this enzyme to stable ring-opened analogues **1** and **1a–1b**, and **1h–1j**, respectively, the related conjugated scaffolds **3** and **4** were fully transformed to highly reactive Michael acceptors that underwent complete transformation to **1c–1g**, and **1k–1n**, respectively.

As members of the aplysinopsin family of marine natural product are long known for their biological properties (i.e., anticancer, antibiotic, antidepressant, antimalarial, and antimicrobial properties) [11], the realisation that they are possible substrates for indoleamine 2,3-dioxygenases is significant. With human indoleamine 2,3-dioxygenase upregulated in key human tissues (i.e., small intestine and lung), and a number of cancers (i.e., acute myeloid leukemia, ovarian, and colorectal carcinoma), knowledge that aplysinopsins are substrates, and yield potent Michael acceptors, could inform future development of this pharmacophore. For example, one might take advantage of the tissue selective abundance of human indoleamine 2,3-dioxygenases for in situ production of highly reactive Michael acceptors (i.e., as warheads within cancer cells). Alternatively, one might seek to diminish the susceptibility of aplysinopsin chemotherapeutics to indoleamine 2,3-dioxygenases, to improve in vivo pharmacokinetics. Either way, an understanding of the biotransformation of aplysinopsins to thorectandrins and spiroreticulatine, and the Michael acceptor status of key intermediates, would inform researchers seeking to exploit the therapeutic potential of these closely related and uniquely marine pharmacophores.

4. Materials and Methods

4.1. General Experimental Procedures

Chiroptical measurements ($[\alpha]_D$) were obtained on a JASCO P-1010 polarimeter (JASCO International Co. Ltd., Tokyo, Japan) in a 100 × 2 mm cell at 23 °C. Electronic Circular Dichroism (ECD) measurement were obtained on a JASCO J-810 spectropolarimeter (JASCO International Co. Ltd., Tokyo, Japan) in a 0.1 cm path-length cell. Nuclear magnetic resonance (NMR) spectra were acquired on a Bruker Avance 600 MHz spectrometer (Bruker Pty. Ltd., Alexandria, Australia) with a 5 mm PASEL ^{1}H/D-^{13}C Z-Gradient probe at 25 °C in methanol-d_4 by referencing to residual ^{1}H or ^{13}C signals (δ_H 3.30 and δ_C 49.15). High-resolution ESIMS spectra were obtained on a Bruker micrOTOF mass spectrometer (Bruker Daltonik Pty. Ltd., Preston, Australia) by direct injection in MeOH at 3 µL/min, using sodium formate clusters as an internal calibrant. Semi-preparative HPLC was performed using Agilent 1100 series HPLC instrument (Agilent Technologies Inc., Mulgrave, Australia) with corresponding detector, fraction collector and software inclusively. Analytical-grade solvents were used for extractions and partitions. Chromatography solvents were of HPLC grade and filtered/degassed through 0.45 µm polytetrafluoroethylene (PTFE) membrane prior to use. Deuterated solvents were purchased from Cambridge Isotopes (Cambridge Isotope Laboratories, Tewksbury, MA, USA). The human colorectal (SW620) and lung

(NCI-H460) carcinoma cell lines were kindly provided by Susan E. Bates and Robert W. Robey of the National Cancer Institute, Bethesda, MD, USA.

4.2. Collection and Taxonomy

Sponge specimen CMB-01889 was collected in July 1995 using epibenthic sled (RV Franklin vessel) at a depth of 45 m in the Great Australian Bight. The specimen was immediately frozen and transported at 0 °C to the laboratory, where it was thawed, documented, diced, and stored in EtOH, at −30 °C prior to chemical investigation. The specimen was taxonomically classified as a *Thorectandra choanoides* (Class Demospongiae, Order Dictyoceratida, Family Thorectidae).

4.3. Extraction and Fractionation

An aliquot (60 mL) of the EtOH crude extract was decanted, concentrated in vacuo, and partitioned between *n*-BuOH (20 mL) and H_2O (20 mL) (Figure S3). MS analysis of the partitions indicated localization of the target GNPS cluster in the *n*-BuOH partition. The *n*-BuOH soluble material was dissolved in MeOH and subjected to HPLC fractionation (Agilent Zorbax SB-CN 9.4 × 250 mm, 5 µm, 3 mL/min gradient elution over 25 min from 10% MeCN/H_2O to 60% MeCN/H_2O, with constant 0.01% TFA modifier), to yield thorectandrin A (**1**) (t_R = 15.2 min, 1.2 mg, 0.6%) (Figure S4).

4.4. Global Natural Product Social (GNPS) Molecular Networking

Aliquots (10 µL) of the *n*-BuOH soluble stock plates prepared from 980 Southern Australian marine sponges were dispensed into 96-well plates, dried under N_2 gas, resuspended in DMSO (10 µL). A total of 0.1 µL of DMSO aliquot was injected into an Agilent 6545 QTOF LC/MS (Agilent Technologies Inc., Mulgrave, Australia) equipped with an Agilent 1290 infinity II UHPLC system, utilizing an Agilent SB-C_8 1.8 µm, 2.1 × 50 mm column, with a 0.5 mL/min, 4.5 min gradient elution from 90% H_2O/MeCN to 100% MeCN, followed by isocratic elution with 100% MeCN for 1 min, with a constant isocratic 0.1% formic acid modifier. The UPLC-QTOF-(+)MS/MS (Agilent Technologies Inc., Mulgrave, Australia) data were acquired for all samples at a fixed collision energy of 40 eV, converted from Agilent MassHunter data files (.d) to mzXML file format, and transferred to the GNPS server (gnps.ucsd.edu) [17]. The full MS/MS data of the 980 sponge extracts could be accessed (accessed on 20 December 2020) from ftp://massive.ucsd.edu/MSV000086621/. Molecular networking was performed using the GNPS data analysis workflow using the spectral clustering algorithm, and a cosine score of 0.7 and a minimum of 6 matched peaks. The resulting spectral networks were visualized using Cytoscape version 3.5.1 (open source software, https://cytoscape.org (accessed on 20 December 2020)) [18], where nodes represented parent *m/z* and edge thickness corresponded to cosine scores, which showed a network featuring ~43,000 nodes, and many hundreds of clusters (Figure S1). Careful review of this GNPS data highlighted a promising cluster (Figure S2) with possible new compounds, associated uniquely with only one sponge specimen, CMB-01889.

4.5. Metabolite Characterization

Thorectandrin A (**1**): light yellow oil; $[\alpha]_D^{22.6}$ 0 (*c* 0.08, MeOH); NMR (methanol-d_4), Table 1 and Figures S5–S10. HRESIMS *m/z* 339.0460/341.0454 [M + H]$^+$ (calculated for $C_{13}H_{16}^{79}BrN_4O_2$, 339.0451; $C_{13}H_{16}^{81}BrN_4O_2$, 341.0431).

Supplementary Materials: The following are available online at https://www.mdpi.com/1660-3397/19/2/97/s1. Full GNPS molecular network, isolation scheme and HPLC chromatogram, 1D and 2D NMR spectra, and HRMS spectrum and bioassay protocols.

Author Contributions: R.J.C. conceptualized the research and assembled the marine sponge collection; S.K. performed dereplication and GNPS analyses, carried out the isolation and spectroscopic characterization of thorectandrin A; L.N. performed bioassays; A.H.E. acquired ECD spectrum; A.A.S. and S.K. constructed the Supplementary Materials document; R.J.C. reviewed all data and drafted the manuscript, with support from S.K. and A.A.S. All authors have read and agreed to the published version of the manuscript.

Funding: This research was supported in part by The University of Queensland and the Institute for Molecular Bioscience.

Institutional Review Board Statement: Not applicable.

Informed Consent Statement: Not applicable.

Data Availability Statement: The full MS/MS data of the 980 sponge extracts could be accessed from ftp://massive.ucsd.edu/MSV000086621/.

Acknowledgments: We thank L Goudie for sponge identification and Z Khalil for bioassays support. S.K., A.H.E. and L.N. acknowledge The University of Queensland for international postgraduate scholarships.

Conflicts of Interest: The authors declare no conflict of interest.

References

1. Cambie, R.C.; Craw, P.A. Chemistry of Sponges, III. Manoalide Monoacetate and Thorectolide Monoacetate, Two New Sesterterpenoids from *Thorectandra excavatus*. *J. Nat. Prod.* **1988**, *51*, 331–334. [CrossRef]
2. Urban, S.; Capon, R.J. A New Furanoditerpene from a Southern Australian Marine Sponge, *Thorectandra choanoides*. *Aust. J. Chem.* **1995**, *48*, 1903–1906. [CrossRef]
3. Charan, R.D.; McKee, T.C.; Boyd, M.R. Thorectandrols A and B, New Cytotoxic Sesterterpenes from the Marine Sponge *Thorectandra* Species. *J. Nat. Prod.* **2001**, *64*, 661–663. [CrossRef]
4. Charan, R.D.; McKee, T.C.; Boyd, M.R. Thorectandrols C, D, and E, New Sesterterpenes from the Marine Sponge *Thorectandra* sp. *J. Nat. Prod.* **2002**, *65*, 492–495. [CrossRef]
5. Charan, R.D.; McKee, T.C.; Gustafson, K.R.; Pannell, L.K.; Boyd, M.R. Thorectandramine, a novel β-carboline alkaloid from the marine sponge *Thorectandra* sp. *Tetrahedron Lett.* **2002**, *43*, 5201–5204. [CrossRef]
6. Charan, R.D.; McKee, T.C.; Boyd, M.R. Cytotoxic Alkaloids from the Marine Sponge *Thorectandra* sp. *Nat. Prod. Res.* **2004**, *18*, 225–229. [CrossRef] [PubMed]
7. Segraves, N.L.; Crews, P. Investigation of Brominated Tryptophan Alkaloids from Two Thorectidae Sponges: *Thorectandra* and *Smenospongia*. *J. Nat. Prod.* **2005**, *68*, 1484–1488. [CrossRef] [PubMed]
8. Khushi, S.; Nahar, L.; Salim, A.A.; Capon, R.J. Trachycladindoles H–M: Molecular Networking Guided Exploration of a Library of Southern Australian Marine Sponges. *Aust. J. Chem.* **2020**, *73*, 338. [CrossRef]
9. Khushi, S.; Nahar, L.; Salim, A.; Capon, R. Cacolides: Sesterterpene Butenolides from a Southern Australian Marine Sponge, *Cacospongia* sp. *Mar. Drugs* **2018**, *16*, 456. [CrossRef]
10. Khushi, S.; Salim, A.A.; Elbanna, A.H.; Nahar, L.; Bernhardt, P.V.; Capon, R.J. Dysidealactams and Dysidealactones: Sesquiterpene Glycinyl- Lactams, Imides, and Lactones from a *Dysidea* sp. Marine Sponge Collected in Southern Australia. *J. Nat. Prod.* **2020**, *83*, 1577–1584. [CrossRef] [PubMed]
11. Bialonska, D.; Zjawiony, J. Aplysinopsins—Marine Indole Alkaloids: Chemistry, Bioactivity and Ecological Significance. *Mar. Drugs* **2009**, *7*, 166–183. [CrossRef] [PubMed]
12. Botting, N.P. Chemistry and neurochemistry of the kynurenine pathway of tryptophan metabolism. *Chem. Soc. Rev.* **1995**, *24*, 401–412. [CrossRef]
13. Wang, Q.; Tang, X.; Luo, X.; Voogd, N.J.; Li, P.; Li, G. (+)- and (−)-Spiroreticulatine, A Pair of Unusual Spiro Bisheterocyclic Quinoline-imidazole Alkaloids from the South China Sea Sponge *Fascaplysinopsis reticulata*. *Org. Lett.* **2015**, *17*, 3458–3461. [CrossRef] [PubMed]
14. Wang, Q.; Tang, X.; Luo, X.; Voogd, N.J.; Li, P.; Li, G. Aplysinopsin-type and Bromotyrosine-derived Alkaloids from the South China Sea Sponge *Fascaplysinopsis reticulata*. *Sci. Rep.* **2019**, *9*, 2248. [CrossRef]
15. Capon, R.J. Extracting value: Mechanistic insights into the formation of natural product artifacts—Case studies in marine natural products. *Nat. Prod. Rep.* **2020**, *37*, 55–79. [CrossRef]
16. Kazlauskas, R.; Murphy, P.T.; Quinn, R.J.; Wells, R.J. Aplysinopsin, a new tryptophan derivative from a sponge. *Tetrahedron Lett.* **1977**, *1*, 61–64. [CrossRef]
17. Wang, M.; Carver, J.J.; Phelan, V.V.; Sanchez, L.M.; Garg, N.; Peng, Y.; Nguyen, D.D.; Watrous, J.; Kapono, C.A.; Luzzatto-Knaan, T.; et al. Sharing and community curation of mass spectrometry data with GNPS. *Nat. Biotechnol.* **2016**, *34*, 828–837. [CrossRef] [PubMed]
18. Shannon, P.; Markiel, A.; Ozier, O.; Baliga, N.S.; Wang, J.T.; Ramage, D.; Amin, N.; Schwikowski, B.; Ideker, T. Cytoscape: A Software Environment for Integrated Models of Biomolecular Interaction Networks. *Genome Res.* **2003**, *13*, 2498–2504. [CrossRef]

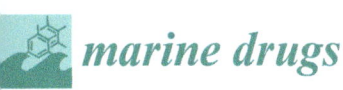

Review

Cellular Signal Transductions and Their Inhibitors Derived from Deep-Sea Organisms

Liyan Wang [1] and Kazuo Umezawa [2,*]

[1] Shenzhen Key Laboratory of Marine Bioresource and Eco-Environmental Science, College of Life Sciences and Oceanography, Shenzhen University, Shenzhen 518060, China; lwang@szu.edu.cn
[2] Molecular Target Medicine, School of Medicine, Aichi Medical University, Nagakute 480-1195, Japan
* Correspondence: umezawa@aichi-med-u.ac.jp; Tel.: +81-561-611-959

Abstract: Not only physiological phenomena but also pathological phenomena can now be explained by the change of signal transduction in the cells of specific tissues. Commonly used cellular signal transductions are limited. They consist of the protein–tyrosine kinase dependent or independent Ras-ERK pathway, and the PI3K-Akt, JAK-STAT, SMAD, and NF-κB-activation pathways. In addition, biodegradation systems, such as the ubiquitin–proteasome pathway and autophagy, are also important for physiological and pathological conditions. If we can control signaling for each by a low-molecular-weight agent, it would be possible to treat diseases in new ways. At present, such cell signaling inhibitors are mainly looked for in plants, soil microorganisms, and the chemical library. The screening of bioactive metabolites from deep-sea organisms should be valuable because of the high incidence of finding novel compounds. Although it is still an emerging field, there are many successful examples, with new cell signaling inhibitors. In this review, we would like to explain the current view of the cell signaling systems important in diseases, and show the inhibitors found from deep-sea organisms, with their structures and biological activities. These inhibitors are possible candidates for anti-inflammatory agents, modulators of metabolic syndromes, antimicrobial agents, and anticancer agents.

Keywords: cellular signal transduction; bioactive metabolite; deep-sea organisms; anti-inflammatory agent; anticancer agent

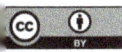

1. Introduction

Nowadays most pathological phenomena such as inflammation, cancer, and diabetes mellitus can be explained by a change of signal transduction in the cells of specific tissues. Therefore, if we could control the specific signal transductions in the body, it would be possible to ameliorate diseases using new concepts. There are several ways to control cellular signal transductions; they are gene-editing therapy; protein therapy, such as providing antibodies or growth factors; and chemotherapy using low molecular weight compounds. Among them, chemotherapy has several advantages, because it is ready to use and free from ethical problems and unwanted immunity. Moreover, signal transduction inhibitors of low molecular weight can be screened similarly to antibiotics, anticancer agents, and enzyme inhibitors from nature.

In the present review, we explain signal transductions in relation to diseases, the methodology of inhibitor screening, screening sources past and present, and finally, we describe examples of the isolation of cell signaling inhibitors from deep-sea organisms.

2. Cellular Signal Transduction and Alteration in Disease

Cyclic AMP was discovered by Sutherland in the 1950s and was called a "second messenger" [1]. Since then, many second messengers that are intracellular signaling transducers have been found. A typical image of a signal transduction from the extracellular ligand to transcription factors is shown in Figure 1A. The signaling molecules shown by the arrow are enzymes or signaling molecules without enzyme activity. The most common signal transductions for the activity of various ligands, hormones, and growth factors are shown in Figure 1B. It is interesting that only a limited number of signaling pathways are commonly used for most activities in the body, even though there are large numbers of tissues, cell types, and functions.

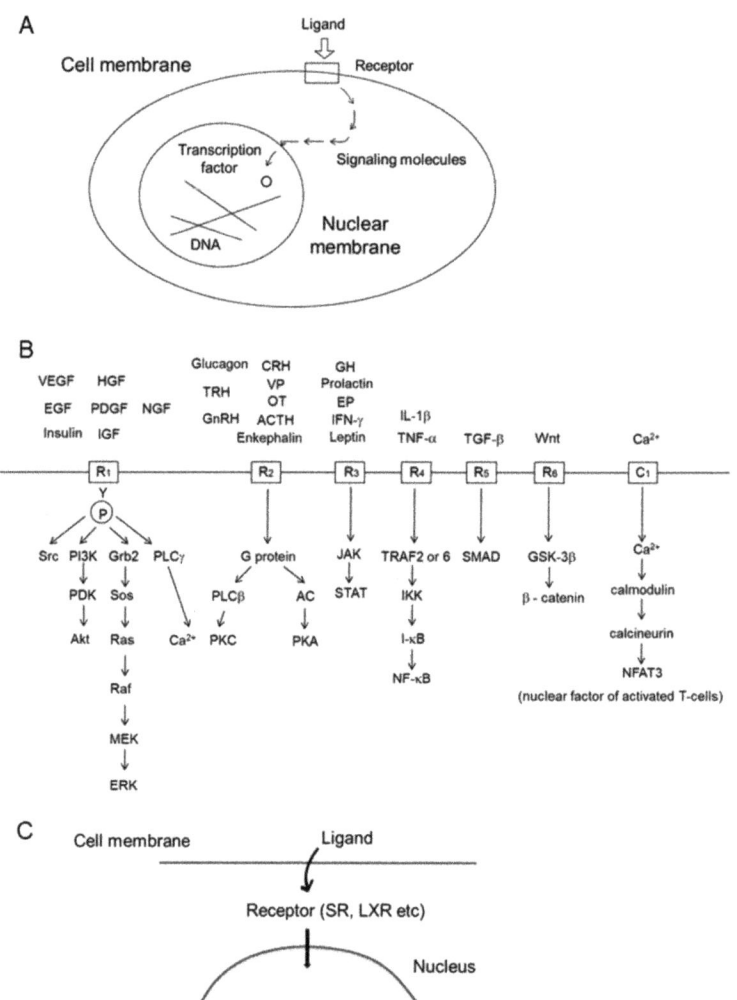

Figure 1. Cellular signal transduction pathways. (**A**) Image of intracellular signal transduction. (**B**) Typical signal transduction pathways commonly used in the cell. (**C**) Intracellular signaling via cytoplasmic receptors. SR, steroid receptor; LXR, liver X receptor.

Many growth factors, such as PDGF, EGF, VEGF, HGF, and IGF, bind to the cell surface receptors having protein–tyrosine kinase to activate the Ras-ERK and PI3K-Akt pathways (Figure 1B, R_1). The growth promoting Ras-ERK pathway and apoptosis-inhibiting PI3K-Akt pathway are considered to be suitable targets for anticancer agents. Both the surface receptor-type, and cytoplasmic type, of protein–tyrosine kinases are associated with many oncogene products. We isolated a novel protein–tyrosine kinase inhibitor, lavendustin, from *Streptomyces* [2]. Bcr-Abl protein–tyrosine kinase is a cytoplasmic type, and the enzyme activity is activated in chronic myelogenous leukemia. Its inhibitor, imatinib, is a successful example of a signal transduction inhibitor that has been developed as orally active anticancer agent against chronic myelogenous leukemia [3]. Protein–tyrosine phosphatase (PTPase) is an opposite enzyme of protein–tyrosine kinase, and known to weaken the insulin-dependent signal transduction. Therefore, its inhibitors may become drugs for type 2 diabetes mellitus. We isolated the first naturally occurring PTPase inhibitor, dephostatin, from *Streptomyces* [4], and its designed analog was shown to inhibit PTP-1B and lower blood glucose in vivo [5].

Receptors of many amino acids or peptide hormones, such as adrenalin, glucagon, vasopressin (VP), oxytocin (OX), gonadotropin releasing hormone (GnRH), ACTH, and enkephalin, activate receptors (Figure 1B, R_2) to activate either cyclic AMP production or phospholipase C activity. This cyclic AMP pathway was discovered by Sutherland [1].

Receptors of growth hormone (GH), erythropoietin (EP), and obesity-preventing leptin (Figure 1B, R_3) do not possess protein–tyrosine kinase, but they activate the kinase activity of JAK in order to activate the STAT transcription factor activity.

TNF-α, interleukin (IL)-1β, and lipopolysaccharide (LPS) bind to the receptors that activate NF-κB (Figure 1B, R_4). Typically, each receptor activates either TRAF6 or TRAF2, which then activates I-κB kinase (IKK) to facilitate the degradation of endogenous inhibitor I-κB by the ubiquitin/proteasome system. NF-κB is a transcription factor that enhances expressions of many inflammatory cytokines and anti-apoptosis proteins. NF-κB is often over-activated in tissue with inflammation and also in cancer cells. Therefore, NF-κB is an attractive target for chemotherapeutic agents, although it is also essential for physiological processes such as blood cell differentiation. The TNF-α antibody is now being used for anti-inflammatory therapy in rheumatoid arthritis and inflammatory bowel disease. Dehydroxymethylepoxyquinomicin (DHMEQ) was discovered by one of the authors as a specific inhibitor of NF-κB. It is a designed compound based on the structure of weak but non-toxic antibiotic epoxyquinomicin [6,7]. It is being developed as an anti-inflammatory ointment for atopic dermatitis and severe skin inflammation [8]. Avoiding the side effects of NF-κB inhibitors, DHMEQ intraperitoneal therapy is being developed for the suppression of cancer [9].

TGF-β binds to cell surface receptors (Figure 1B, R_5) to activate SMAD proteins acting as transcription factors. It often induces fibrosis in the liver, lungs, pancreas, and peritoneal cavity. TGF-β also accelerates the epidermal mesenchymal transition (EMT) that enhances malignancy in cancer cells [10]. We found that the plant-derived alkaloid conophylline inhibited TGF-β receptor downstream signaling [11].

The Wnt/β-catenin pathway is often activated in cancer cells. In this pathway, stimulation of the receptor by the Wnt ligand (Figure 1B, R_6) activates GSK-3β to activate β-catenin. Aggregated β-catenins enter into the nucleus to act as a transcription factor together with the TCF–LEF complex.

The calcineurin–NFAT pathway was discovered by a chemical biology technique using a fishing probe of immune-suppressant FK506 (tacrolimus) derivative [12]. After the incorporation of calcium ions through the calcium channel (Figure 1B,C), calcium ion-dependent calmodulin activates calcineurin to activate the nuclear factor of activated T-cells-3 (NFAT3). FK506 and cyclosporine inactivate calcineurin through their binding proteins.

Steroid hormones are lipophilic and can pass through the cell membrane (Figure 1C). Their receptors exist in the cytoplasm and after binding the ligand-receptor complex enter the nucleus to bind to the promoter site of DNA, acting as a transcription factor. Liver X receptors also exist in the cytoplasm and their ligands bind to the receptor there to enter the nucleus.

In addition to the signal transductions in Figure 1B,C, there are two protein degradation pathways that have been recently developed. The ubiquitin–proteasome pathway is important for the regulation of cellular signal transduction [13]. For example, activation of NF-κB requires degradation of inhibitory protein I-κB, and the degradation is carried out by proteasomes after ubiquitination (Figure 2A). Bortezomib is an inhibitor of proteasomes and is now being clinically used for the treatment of multiple myeloma [14]. While the ubiquitin–proteasome system is important for the degradation of specific proteins, autophagy is important for the degradation of mass biomaterials. The process of autophagy (Figure 2B) is initiated by the formation of autophagosome during the wrapping of biomaterials by the double membrane system in the cytoplasm [15]. Autophagy is caused by the lysosome-mediated degradation of damaged proteins and organelles, as well as unwanted bacteria and viruses. It is essential for the loss of mitochondria in the evolution of red blood cells and for the cellular antibacterial activity against *Mycobacterium tuberculosis* [16]. The age-dependent decrease in autophagy activity in the brain is considered to accelerate neurodegenerative diseases. We have looked for the activators of cellular autophagy and have previously reported that the plant-derived alkaloid conophylline ameliorated cellular models of Parkinson's and Huntington's diseases by the activation of autophagy [17]. Conophylline also activated autophagy in the liver of high fat diet-induced non-alcoholic steatohepatitis (NASH) mice [18]. Although molecular targets for the screening of autophagy activators or inhibitors are not yet clear, it would be useful to look for the non-toxic regulator of autophagy.

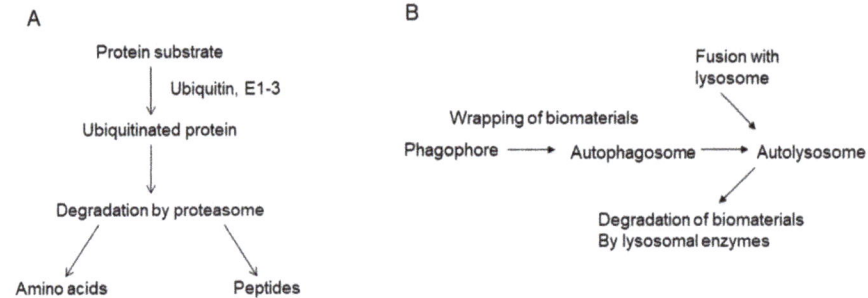

Figure 2. Protein degradation systems. (**A**) Ubiquitin–proteasome biodegradation system. (**B**) Process of autophagy.

Thus, not only the physiological role of tissues and cells, but also the mechanism of diseases can be explained by changes of signal transductions, mostly shown in Figures 1 and 2. The chemical inhibitors of cellular signal transduction, which is over-activated in the cells or tissues in diseases, should be useful as a rational drug for each disease.

3. Process of Screening and Deep-Sea Organisms as a Source of Bioactive Metabolites

The process of bioactive metabolite screening we employed is shown in Figure 3A. Setting up a biological assay system is the most important process. The biological assay systems include antibacterial activity, measurement of enzyme activity, and cellular morphology, growth, apoptosis, and differentiation. The biological activity should reflect the essential signal transduction in diseases. In the case of drug screening, if the activity is not essential for the etiology of disease, the screened signaling inhibitor will be useless in further disease models or at the clinical stage. The biological activity should be simple and carried out economically and effectively. The enzyme assay and cellular assay are the most popular for screening.

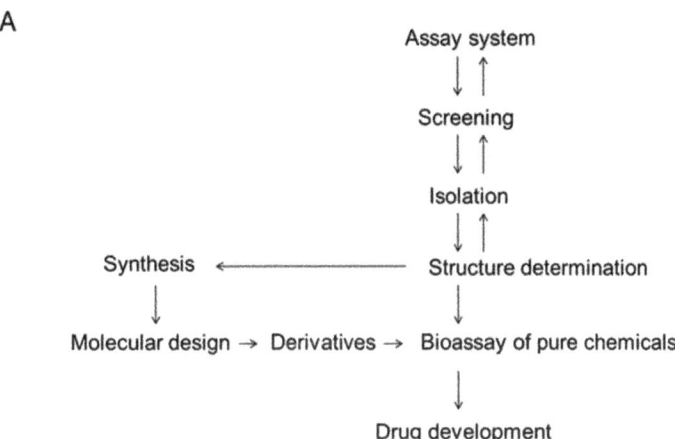

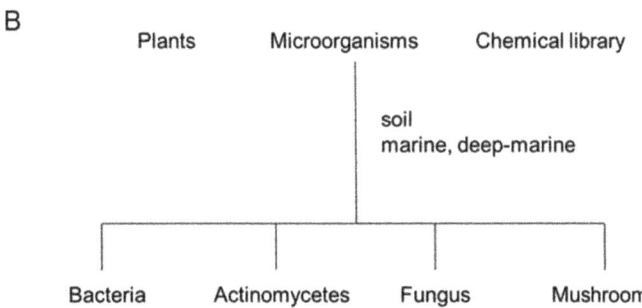

Figure 3. Screening of bioactive metabolites. (**A**) Process of natural product screening. (**B**) Screening sources.

After the screening of plants or microorganisms to find a hit, we began isolation using various chromatography techniques and structure determination by spectroscopy, including nuclear magnetic resonance and mass spectrometry. After determining the structure, we studied the effect of signal transduction inhibitors on various biological activities, including the cellular and animal toxicity. If it is possible, the compound is synthesized to facilitate enough supply and derivative preparation. If the original or derivative compound suppresses the disease models satisfactorily, we will try to develop it into a drug together with the industry. Meanwhile, we have been studying the mechanism of diseases using the signal transduction inhibitors in cultured cells or animal experiments.

Secondary metabolites are defined as low-molecular weight compounds produced by biological organisms that are not essential for the life of the producers. Secondary metabolites are produced only by plants and microorganisms. Tetrodotoxin is produced by fish and many secondary metabolites are produced by sponges. However, these compounds are considered to be produced by parasitic microorganisms. Bioactive metabolites are secondary metabolites that possess specific biological activities. The specific biological activity should be shown at comparatively low concentrations or doses.

Penicillin was isolated from a fungus, *Penicillium notatum*, and streptomycin from *Streptomyces griseus*, in the 1940s. Since then, many antibiotics, anticancer drugs, and enzyme inhibitors have been isolated from microorganisms and plants. Microorganisms and plants are still useful sources for the screening of useful drugs. Natural sources of signal transduction inhibitors are summarized in Figure 3B.

Many scientists have tried to isolate novel compounds from plants, soil microorganisms (including bacteria, *Streptomyces*, and fungi), and ordinary marine organisms since the middle of the 20th century. However, after a long history of screening, it is getting more difficult to find novel compounds anywhere in the world.

Meanwhile, more than 28,600 marine natural products have been reported. However, with the development of marine natural product research, the hit rate of new compounds is decreasing. Therefore, scientists are turning their attention to the deep sea. By 2008, almost 400 compounds were isolated from deep-sea organisms. By 2013, a further 188 new deep-sea natural products had been reported. About 75% of compounds from such an origin were reported to show biological activity (i.e., 141 of 188 compounds), with almost half (i.e., 81 of 188 compounds) exhibiting potent cytotoxicity in human cancer cell lines [19]. Blunt reported the effective screening of cytotoxic compounds with double the frequency from a single deep-water collection in New Zealand, compared with that of shallow water collections [20].

Sponges, corals, and fish also produce bioactive metabolites, although these metabolites are considered to be produced by parasitic microorganisms. In addition to the microorganisms, there are also sponges and corals in the deep sea. An investigation of the extracts of 65 "twilight zone" (50–1000 m depth) sponges, gorgonians, hard corals, and sponge-associated bacteria resulted in an extremely high hit rate (42%) of active extracts, with that for sponge and gorgonian extracts being 72% [21,22]. Thus, deep-sea organisms are considered to be important sources of natural products, especially for the screening of new cell signaling inhibitors.

4. Anti-Inflammatory Agents from Deep-Sea Organisms

4.1. Cyclopenol and Cyclopenin Inhibiting NF-κB Signaling

In the course of screening lipopolysaccharide (LPS)-induced nitric oxide (NO) production inhibitors, two related benzodiazepine derivatives, cyclopenol and cyclopenin (Figure 4), were isolated from the extract of a fungal strain, *Aspergillus* sp. SCSIOW2 [23]. The fungus was isolated from a deep marine sediment sample collected in the South China Sea at a depth of 2439 m. Cyclopenin was first isolated and reported in 1954 from a strain of *Penicillium cyclopium* [24], and cyclopenol was then isolated in 1963 from the same strain [25]. Cyclopenol and cyclopenin inhibited the LPS-induced formation of NO and secretion of interleukin-6 (IL-6) in RAW264.7 cells at non-toxic concentrations. In terms of the mechanism underlying these effects, cyclopenol and cyclopenin were found to inhibit the upstream signal of NF-κB activation.

Microglia are located in the brain for cleaning and protection against microorganisms, acting as macrophages in the brain. The 6-1 mouse microglia cell line was established and used to examine whether cyclopenol and cyclopenin inhibit LPS-induced inflammatory mediator protein expression in microglia. The results revealed that both clearly inhibited the expression of interleukin-1β (IL-1β), IL-6, and inducible NO synthase (iNOS).

Finally, the anti-inflammatory effects of cyclopenol and cyclopenin were examined in vivo. The ameliorative effect on learning deficits was assessed using amyloid-β-overexpressing *Drosophylla* flies, since only a small quantity of sample was necessary in this assay. Memantine, a derivative of adamantane, is an NMDA receptor antagonist clinically used for the treatment of Alzheimer's disease. Memantine was used as the positive control. We found that cyclopenin rescued learning impairment, similar to memantine [23]. By contrast, cyclopenol did not ameliorate learning activity impairment. The hydroxyl group in cyclopenol may reduce the permeability of the compound and would make penetration into the body difficult.

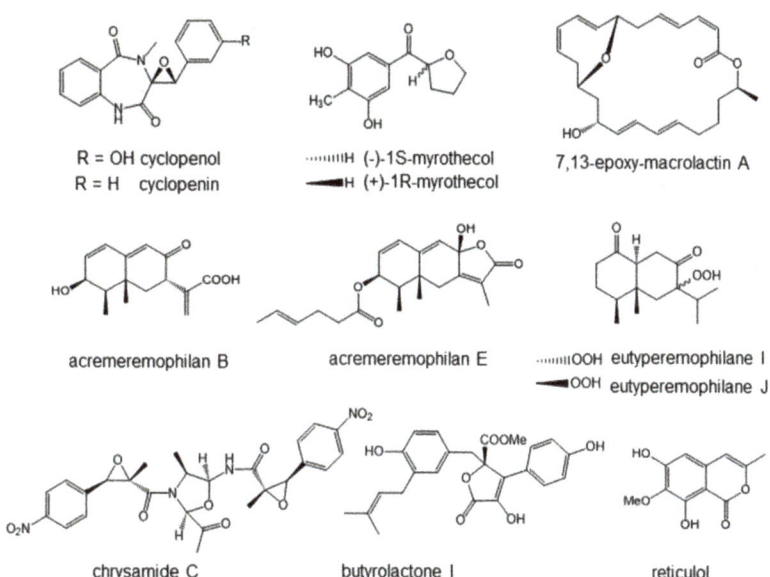

Figure 4. Anti-inflammatory agents isolated from deep-sea organisms.

4.2. Myrothenols Inhibiting LPS-Induced NO Production

We recently looked for novel compounds having anti-inflammatory activity from deep-sea microorganisms. As a result, we have isolated four new compounds, a pair of 2-benzoyl tetrahydrofuran enantiomers, named (−)-1S-myrothecol (Figure 4), (+)-1R-myrothecol (Figure 4), methoxy-myrothecol, and an azaphilone derivative, myrothin, from the culture filtrates of the deep sea-derived fungus, *Myrothecium* sp. BZO-L062 [26]. The fungus was isolated from a deep marine (2130 m deep) sediment sample, collected from an area close to Yongxing Island, China. The enantiomeric (−)-1S- and (+)-1R-myrothecol were separated by chiral normal phase high performance liquid chromatography (HPLC). Among all the isolated compounds, (−)-1S- and (+)-1R-myrothecol showed cellular anti-inflammatory activity inhibiting NO formation in LPS-treated macrophage-like cells.

LPS-induced NO production in mouse monocytic leukemia RAW264.7 cells, which are often employed for the evaluation of cellular anti-inflammatory activity because of similarities in phenotypes with macrophages. Both (−)-1S- and (+)-1R-myrothecol inhibited the LPS-induced NO production at non-toxic concentrations. The mechanism of inhibition remains to be elucidated.

Anti-oxidant activities can be measured by oxygen radical absorbance capacity (ORAC) assay. Both (−)-1S- and (+)-1R-myrothecol showed an antioxidant activity in the ORAC assay, with EC_{50} of 1.20 and 1.41 µg/mL, respectively, which were comparable with the positive controls, L-ascorbic acid (EC_{50}, 1.55 µg/mL) and trolox (EC_{50}, 1.61 µg/mL).

4.3. Macrolactins Inhibiting NO and Cytokine Productions

Novel macrolactin, 7,13-epoxyl-macrolactin A (Figure 4), was isolated from deep-sea sediment as an inhibitor of LPS-induced inflammatory mediator expression in RAW264.7 cells [27]. The producing strain was isolated from sediment collected at a depth of 3000 m in the Pacific Ocean, and identified as *Bacillus subtilis* B5 by the complete 16S rRNA gene sequence. This new macrolactin exhibited a more potent inhibitory effect on NO production and several inflammatory cytokines than the previously known macrolactins, such as macrolactin A and analogues. Macrolactin A also inhibited the mRNA expression of iNOS, IL-1β, and IL-6 in LPS-stimulated RAW 264.7 cells.

4.4. Acremeremophilanes Inhibiting LPS-Induced NO Production

Separation and structural determination of an EtOAc extract of the culture filtrate of the fungus, *Acremonium* sp., from deep-sea sediment, resulted in the isolation of 15 new eremophilane-type sesquiterpenoids, acremeremophilanes A–O [28]. The fungus was collected from sediment at a depth of 2869 m in the South Atlantic Ocean.

All compounds were evaluated for inhibitory effects toward LPS-induced NO production in RAW 264.7 cells. Among them, acremeremophilane B (EC_{50}, 8 µM, Figure 4) and E (EC_{50}, 15 µM, Figure 4) showed comparatively potent inhibitory activities at non-toxic concentrations. A positive control, quercetin, inhibited NO production with EC_{50} of 15 µM in this system. The mechanism of inhibition remains to be elucidated.

4.5. Eutyperemophilanes Inhibiting LPS-Induced NO Production

Anti-inflammatory agents were searched for in the manipulated deep-sea microorganisms. The fungus, *Eutypella* sp. MCCC 3A00281, was collected from sediment at the extreme depth of 5610 m in the South Atlantic Ocean. Cultivation of the fungus by chemical epigenetic manipulation using suberohydroxamic acid, a histone deacetylase inhibitor, resulted in a significant change in the metabolite profile. Chromatographic application of the extended metabolites led to the isolation of a total of 30 eremophilane-type sesquiterpenoids, of which 26 were identified as new compounds, namely eutyperemophilanes A–Z [29]. All the compounds were evaluated for inhibitory effects on LPS-induced NO production in RAW264.7 cells. Among the 30 compounds, eutyperemophilane I and J (Figure 4) showed comparatively potent inhibition with IC_{50} of 8.6 and 13 µM, respectively (positive control quercetin, 16 µM), all at nontoxic concentrations.

4.6. Chrysamide C Inhibiting Interleukin-17 Production

Three dimeric nitrophenyl trans-epoxyamides, chrysamides A–C, were obtained from the deep-sea-derived fungus, *Penicillium chrysogenum* SCSIO41001 [30]. The fungal strain used was isolated from deep-sea sediment from the Indian Ocean at a depth of 3386 m. These compounds showed cytotoxicity at 30 µM in cancer cells. Chrysamide C (Figure 4) only possessed the oxazolidine ring, differentiating it from chrysamide A and B. Chrysamide C, but not A and B, suppressed the production of proinflammatory cytokine interleukin-17 (IL-17). The inhibitory rate on the production of IL-17 was 40.06% at 1.0 µM, while the rate of the positive control SR2211 was 62.86% at 1.0 µM. For the evaluation of IL-17 production, naive T-cells were isolated from IL-17-GFP reporter mice spleen, and then stimulated with anti-CD3, anti-CD28, TGF-β, IL-6, anti-IFN-γ, and anti-IL-4 in the presence of test chemicals. IL-17 is mainly produced by activated T-lymphocytes, and induces inflammatory cytokine and chemokine secretions in fibroblasts, epithelial cells, endothelial cells, and macrophages.

4.7. Butyrolactone I Suppressing Mast Cell Activity

A food allergy is defined as an immune-mediated adverse reaction to a food. Egg allergy is common in children worldwide and is considered to be mainly caused by ovalbumin. Therefore, ovalbumin is often used to construct animal models of food allergy. A type I allergic reaction is mediated by antigen specific IgE that causes mast cell degranulation [31], and this reaction leads to anaphylactic shock when it takes place in the whole body [32]. Mast cells secrete leukotrienes, histamine, and prostaglandins upon activation with antigen and IgE, and they play a central role in allergic reactions. Allergic inflammation is characterized by the tissue infiltration of inflammatory cells, including mast cells, macrophages, and lymphocytes. For the cellular assay of an allergic reaction, antigen and IGE-responsive rat basophilic leukemia RBL-2H3 cells are often employed [33].

Butyrolactone I (Figure 4), which was identified as a new type of butanolide, was isolated from a deep-sea-derived fungus, *Aspergillus* sp. [34]. The fungus was isolated from a hydrothermal sulfide deposit in the southwest Indian Ocean at a depth of 2783 m.

Ovalbumin-induced BALB/c mouse anaphylaxis model was established to study food allergic activity. Butyrolactone I ameliorated ovalbumin-induced allergy symptoms, and reduced the levels of histamine and mouse mast cell proteinases. It inhibited ovalbumin-caused production of IgE, and inhibited the accumulation of mast cells in the spleen and mesenteric lymph nodes. It also significantly suppressed mast cell-dependent passive cutaneous anaphylaxis. Additionally, the butyrolactone-I caused down-regulation of c-KIT receptors to reduce maturation of mast cells. Moreover, molecular docking analyses revealed that butylolactone I would interact with the inhibitory receptor, FcγRIIB.

4.8. Reticurol Suppressing Mast Cell Activity

The same group carried out screening of bioactive compounds from the hydrothermal fungus, *Graphostroma* sp. MCCC 3A00421 [35]. The fungus was isolated from deep-sea hydrothermal sulfide deposits from the Atlantic Ocean at a depth of 2721 m. Nine new compounds, including graphostrin A, and 19 known polyketides, were isolated. All the isolated compounds were tested for cellular anti-food allergic bioactivity in antigen and IgE-treated RBL-2H3 cells. Among them, reticulol (Figure 4), a known polyketide, effectively decreased the rates of degranulation and histamine release, with IC_{50} values of 13.5 and 13.7 μM, respectively. Reticulol was first isolated by Hamao Umezawa and co-workers from *Streptomyces mobaraensis* in 1977 as an inhibitor of cyclic nucleotide phosphodiesterase [36]. It was later discovered to inhibit topoisomerase I [37] in addition to cyclic nucleotide phosphodiesterase, and was shown to exhibit anticancer activity in vivo [38].

5. Modulators of Metabolic Syndrome Model and Antimicrobial Compounds

5.1. Puniceloids C and D, Liver X Receptor Agonists

Liver X receptors (LXR), including LXRα and LXRβ, are critical modulators of cholesterol and lipid metabolism, inflammatory responses, and innate immunity [39]. LXRs are ligand-activated transcription factors that belong to a family of hormone nuclear receptors (Figure 1C). LXR agonists have been suggested to have a potential use in the treatment of atherosclerosis, diabetes, inflammation, and Alzheimer's disease [40].

Eight novel diketopiperazine-type alkaloids, including four oxepin-containing diketopiperazine-type alkaloids, oxepinamides H–K, and four 4-quinazolinone alkaloids, puniceloids A–D, were isolated from culture broth extracts of the deep-sea-derived fungus, *Aspergillus puniceus* SCSIO z021 [41]. The fungus was isolated from deep-sea sediment collected in the Okinawa Trough at the depth of 1589 m, about 4.7 km away from active hydrothermal vents. For the measurement of LXR agonist activity, human hepatocyte L02 cells were transfected by the LXRα reporter system with luciferase gene. These eight compounds showed significant transcriptional activation of LXRα. Among them, puniceloid C and D (Figure 5) were the most potent, both with EC_{50} values of 1.7 μM.

5.2. Chrysopyrones A and B, Protein–Tyrosine Phosphatase Inhibitors That Ameliorate Diabetes Mellitus Model

Diabetes mellitus is caused by two factors: a decrease in insulin production in the pancreatic islet, and a decrease in insulin sensitivity in the target tissues, such as muscle, fat, and liver. The latter is caused by a reduction of insulin-dependent signaling pathways, including insulin receptor, insulin receptor substrates (IRS), phosphatidylinositol 3-kinase (PI3K), and AKT (also called protein kinase B or serine/threonine kinase 1). The insulin receptor possesses protein–tyrosine kinase activity, and its substrates are the insulin receptor itself and IRS. Tyrosine phosphorylation of these proteins is essential for insulin signal transduction. However, if there is protein–tyrosine phosphatase in the cells, this enzyme removes phosphate from the tyrosine residues to weaken the insulin signal. Therefore, inhibitors of protein–tyrosine phosphatase, especially protein–tyrosine phosphatase-1B (PTP1B), should reactivate the insulin-dependent signaling to show the anti-diabetic activity [5,42].

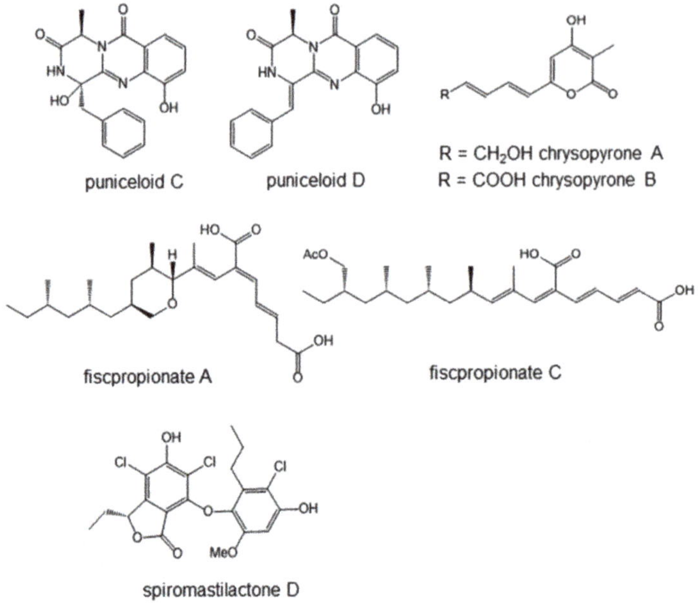

Figure 5. Modulators of metabolic syndrome and antimicrobial compounds isolated from deep-sea organisms.

Two new 3,4,6-trisubstituted α-pyron compounds, chrysopyrones A and B (Figure 5), as well as another new compound, penilline C, and 12 known compounds were isolated from the products of the fungus *Penicillium chrysogenum* SCSIO 07007 [43]. This fungus was separated from deep-sea hydrothermal vent environment samples collected from the western Atlantic at a depth of about 1000 m. Hydrothermal vents are formed through rock fissures located in volcanic regions. Deep-sea hydrothermal vent areas are characterized by high concentrations of reduced sulfur compounds.

Among the isolated compounds, chrysopyrones A and B (Figure 5) inhibited PTP1B with IC_{50} values of 9.32 and 27.8 μg/mL, respectively. They did not show cytotoxicity in cultured cells at 100 μg/mL. Their in vivo anti-diabetic activity remains to be studied.

5.3. Fiscpropionate A and C Inhibiting Bacterial Protein–Tyrosine Phosphatase

It is interesting that protein–tyrosine phosphatase also exists in bacteria and is considered to be the molecular target of antibacterial agents. In particular, *Mycobacterium tuberculosis* protein–tyrosine phosphatase B (MptpB) is an important virulence factor secreted by *Mycobacterium tuberculosis* into the host cell [44,45]. MptpB removes phosphate from the tyrosine residue of host proteins that are involved in the host signaling pathways, and it can attenuate the host immune defenses against tuberculosis. Therefore, MptpB inhibitors can enhance host immunity against *Mycobacterium tuberculosis*.

Fiscpropionates A–F, six new polypropionate derivatives featuring an unusual long hydrophobic chain, were isolated from the deep-sea-derived fungus, *Aspergillus fischeri* FS452 [46]. The fungal strain was isolated from deep-sea sludge in the Indian Ocean at a depth of 3000 m. Fiscpropionates A–D exhibited significant inhibitory activities against MptpB. Among them, fiscpropionates A and C (Figure 5) were comparatively effective, with the IC_{50} values of 5.1 and 4.0 μM, respectively. These compounds may be unique seeds of anti-tuberculosis agents.

5.4. *Spiromastilactone D Inhibits Influenza Virus Replication*

A new class of phenolic lactones with the trivial names of spiromastilactones A–M was isolated from a deep-sea-derived fungus, *Spiromastix* sp. MCCC 3A00308 [47]. The fungus was isolated from sediment collected from the South Atlantic Ocean at a depth of 2869 m. The structures feature varied chlorination of the aromatic rings. An antiviral assay revealed that most of the tested compounds exerted inhibitory activity against influenza virus replication in vitro at nontoxic concentrations. Among them, spiromastilactone D (Figure 5) showed the most potent activity for inhibiting a panel of influenza A and B viruses, in addition to drug-resistant clinical isolates. A mechanistic study using surface plasmon resonance suggested that the molecular target of spiromastilactone D would be hemagglutinin. Hemagglutinin is located in the envelope of the virus, and spiromastilactone D is likely to disrupt the interaction between hemagglutinin and the host sialic acid receptor, which is essential for the attachment and entry of all influenza viruses. In addition, spiromastilactone D showed inhibitory effects toward viral genome replication via targeting viral RNP complex. The synergistic effects on both viral entry and replication indicated it to be a candidate new anti-influenza agent.

6. Anticancer Agents

6.1. *Cytotoxic Agents and Cell Signaling Inhibitors*

Major anticancer drugs such as cisplatin, 5-fuluorouracil (5FU), doxorubicin, vinblastine, and paclitaxel are all cytotoxic compounds. Cisplatin, 5FU, and doxorubicin interact with DNA to inhibit polynucleotide synthesis, while vinblastine and paclitaxel bind to tubulin to inhibit cellular mitosis. These anticancer drugs attack not only cancer cells, but also normal cells, causing side effects. Although several new cytotoxic agents have been isolated from deep-sea organisms, they are not shown in this review. In general, the molecular targets of cytotoxic agents are difficult to find.

Meanwhile, the characteristics of cancer cells include fast growth rate, immortality, less requirement of growth factors, ability for anchorage-independent growth, less contact inhibition of growth, and so on. The selectivity of these anticancer drugs is found only in the fast growth of cancer cells. Generally, these anticancer agents are more effective in suppressing the growth of actively growing cells. Therefore, they damage normal, fast growing cells, such as bone marrow cells, intestine epithelial cells, skin cells, and reproductive organ cells, inducing serious side effects. Imatinib [3] and all-trans retinoic acid (ATRA) [48] are exceptional, since they show anticancer activity through the attack of molecular targets of cancer cells. These molecular target medicines inhibit specific cell signaling pathways.

6.2. *Salinosporamide A, a Proteasome Inhibitor*

The ubiquitin proteasome pathway was discovered in the 1980s, and it is now one of the most important cellular protein-degradation machineries. This pathway is essential for the removal of misfolded proteins, and it is also essential for the regulation of cell cycle and apoptosis [49]. The ubiquitin proteasome pathway down-regulates cell-cycle and tumor-suppressor proteins, such as p21, p27 [50], and p53 [51]. On the other hand, this pathway up-regulates oncogenic proteins, including NF-κB, by the degradation of inhibitory proteins [14]. Bortezomib is a successful example of proteasome inhibitors that are widely used clinically for the treatment of multiple myeloma [14].

Salinosporamide A (Figure 6) was isolated by Fenical et al. in 2003 from the marine actinomycete *Salinispora tropica*, collected at a depth of 1100 m, and it is a highly potent and selective inhibitor of the 20S proteasome [52]. It is a pyrrolidinone compound fused to a beta-lactone, and the structure is partly related to that of lactacystin (Figure 6) [53], an inhibitor of proteasome, isolated from *Streptomyces*. The crystal structure of salinosporamide A-20S proteasome revealed the mechanism of irreversible inhibition with β-lactone ring opening [54].

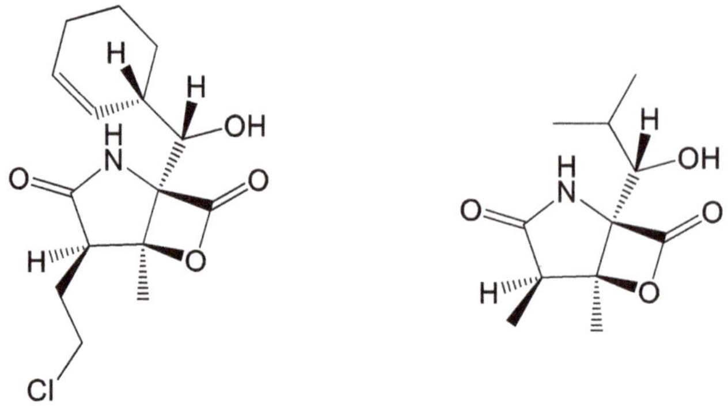

salinosporamide A   **lactacystin A**

Figure 6. Proteasome inhibitors; Salinosporamide A shows anticancer activity.

It suppressed both constitutive and inducible NF-κB activity [55]. Compared with bortezomib and lactacystin, salinosporamide A was found to be the most potent suppressor of NF-κB. Salinosporamide A inhibited I-κBα degradation, nuclear translocation of p65, and NF-κB-dependent gene expression in TNF-α-treated cells, while it showed no effect on I-κB kinase. Clinical trials of salinosporamide A are ongoing for the treatment of multiple myeloma.

7. Conclusions and Perspective

Cell signaling inhibitors from deep-sea organisms are summarized in Table 1.

Table 1. Cell signaling inhibitors isolated from deep-sea organisms.

Natural Products	Target Signal	Related Illustration	Reference
Cyclopenol and cyclopenin	NO production (NF-κB)	Figure 1B, R_4	[23]
Myrothecols	NO production	Figure 1B, R_4	[26]
7,13-Epoxyl-macrolactin A	NO production	Figure 1B, R_4	[27]
Acremeremophilane B	NO production	Figure 1B, R_4	[28]
Eutyperemophilane I and J	NO production	Figure 1B, R_4	[29]
Chrysamide C	IL-17 Production	—*	[30]
Butyrolactone I	Mast cell activity	—	[34]
Reticurol	Mast cell activity	—	[35]
Puniceloids C and D	Liver X receptor	Figure 1C	[41]
Chrysopyrones A and B	Protein–tyrosine phosphatase	Figure 1B, R_1	[43]
Fiscpropionate A and C	Protein–tyrosine phosphatase (bacterial)	—	[46]
Spiromastilactone D	Influenza virus	—	[47]
Salinosporamide A	Proteasome	Figure 2A	[52]

* The mechanism is unknown.

Commonly used cellular signal transductions, such as protein–tyrosine kinase-dependent or independent Ras-ERK pathways and NF-κB-activation pathways, the ubiquitin–proteasome pathway and autophagy, are attractive targets for the discovery of safe, anti-inflammatory and anticancer drugs. At present, such cell signaling inhibitors are being looked for mainly in plants, soil microorganisms, and the chemical library. The screening of bioactive metabolites from deep-sea organisms is attractive because of the high incidence of finding novel compounds. Although it is still an emerging field, there are many successful examples of new cell signaling inhibitors. In particular, a proteasome inhibitor, salinosporamide A, isolated from deep-sea microorganisms is being developed as an anticancer agent. In the future, there are likely to be more cell signaling inhibitors from the deep-sea that will be developed into drugs.

Author Contributions: L.W. and K.U. both contributed to the collection of papers and preparation. All authors have read and agreed to the published version of the manuscript.

Funding: This work was financially supported in part by AMED under Grant Number JP18fk0310118JSPS, Kakenhi Grant Number 17K01967, and Chinese National Key Research and Development Project 2019YFC0312501.

Data Availability Statement: No new data were created or analyzed in this study. Data sharing is not applicable to this article.

Conflicts of Interest: The authors declare no conflict of interest. Department of Molecular Target Medicine to which K.U. belongs is a fund-donated laboratory. It is supported financially by Shenzhen Wanhe Pharmaceutical Company, Shenzhen, China, Meiji Seika Pharma, Tokyo, Japan, Fukuyu Medical Corporation, Nisshin, Japan, and Brunaise Co., Ltd., Nagoya, Japan.

References

1. Rall, T.W.; Sutherland, E.W. Formation of a cyclic adenine ribonucleotide by tissue particles. *J. Biol. Chem.* **1958**, *232*, 1065–1076. [CrossRef]
2. Onoda, T.; Iinuma, H.; Sasaki, Y.; Hamada, M.; Isshiki, K.; Naganawa, H.; Takeuchi, T.; Tatsuta, K.; Umezawa, K. Isolation of a novel tyrosine kinase inhibitor, lavendustin A, from *Streptomyces griseolavendus*. *J. Nat. Prod.* **1989**, *52*, 1252–1257. [CrossRef] [PubMed]
3. Capdeville, R.; Buchdunger, E.; Zimmermann, J.; Matter, A. Glivec (STI571, imatinib), a rationally developed, targeted anticancer drug. *Nat. Rev. Drug Discov.* **2002**, *1*, 493–502. [CrossRef] [PubMed]
4. Imoto, M.; Kakeya, H.; Sawa, T.; Hayashi, C.; Hamada, M.; Takeuchi, T.; Umezawa, K. Dephostasin, a novel protein tyrosine phosphatase inhibitor produced by *Streptomyce* I. Taxonomy, isolation, and characterization. *J. Antibiot.* **1993**, *46*, 1342–1346. [CrossRef]
5. Suzuki, T.; Hiroki, A.; Watanabe, T.; Yamashita, T.; Takei, I.; Umezawa, K. Potentiation of insulin-related signal transduction by a novel protein-tyrosine phosphatase inhibitor, Et-3,4-dephostatin, on cultured 3T3-L1 adipocytes. *J. Biol. Chem.* **2001**, *276*, 27511–27518. [CrossRef]
6. Matsumoto, N.; Ariga, A.; To-e, S.; Nakamura, H.; Agata, N.; Hirano, S.; Inoue, J.; Umezawa, K. Synthesis of NF-κB activation inhibitors derived from epoxyquinomicin C. *Bioorg. Med. Chem. Lett.* **2000**, *10*, 865–869. [CrossRef]
7. Ariga, A.; Namekawa, J.; Matsumoto, N.; Inoue, J.; Umezawa, K. Inhibition of TNF-κ-induced nuclear translocation and activation of NF-B by dehydroxymethyl-epoxyquinomicin. *J. Biol. Chem.* **2002**, *277*, 27625–27630. [CrossRef]
8. He, H.; Gao, X.; Wang, X.; Li, X.; Jiang, X.; Xie, Z.; Ma, K.; Ma, J.; Umezawa, K.; Zhang, Y. Comparison of anti-atopic dermatitis activities between DHMEQ and tacrolimus ointments in mouse model without stratum corneum. *Int. Immunopharm.* **2019**, *71*, 43–51. [CrossRef]
9. Umezawa, K.; Breborowicz, A.; Gantsev, G. Anticancer activity of novel NF-B inhibitor DHMEQ by intraperitoneal administration. *Oncol. Res.* **2020**, *28*, 541–550. [CrossRef]
10. Liu, S.; Ren, J.; Dijke, P.T. Targeting TGFβ signal transduction for cancer therapy. *Signal Transduct. Target. Ther.* **2021**, *6*, 8. [CrossRef]
11. Atsumi, S.; Nagasawa, A.; Koyano, T.; Kowithayakorn, T.; Umezawa, K. Suppression of TGF-β signaling by conophylline via upregulation of c-Jun expression. *Cell. Mol. Life Sci.* **2003**, *60*, 2516–2525. [CrossRef]
12. Liu, J.; Farmer, J.D., Jr.; Lane, W.S.; Friedman, J.; Weissman, I.; Schreiber, S.L. Calcineurin is a common target of cyclophilin-cyclosporin A and FKBP-FK506 complexes. *Cell* **1991**, *65*, 807–815. [CrossRef]
13. Welchman, R.L.; Gordon, C.; Mayer, R.J. Ubiquitin and ubiquitin-like proteins as multifunctional signals. *Nat. Rev. Mol. Cell Biol.* **2005**, *6*, 599–609. [CrossRef]
14. Paramore, F.; Franz, S. Bortezomib. *Nat. Rev. Drug Discov.* **2003**, *2*, 611–612. [CrossRef]
15. Dikic, I.; Elazar, Z. Mechanism and medical implications of mammalian autophagy. *Nat. Rev. Mol. Cell Biol.* **2018**, *19*, 349–364. [CrossRef]
16. Jing, K.; Lim, K. Why is autophagy important in human diseases? *Exp. Mol. Med.* **2012**, *44*, 69–72. [CrossRef]
17. Sasazawa, Y.; Sato, N.; Umezawa, K.; Simizu, S. Conophylline protects cells in cellular models of neurodegenerative diseases by inducing mTOR-independent autophagy. *J. Biol. Chem.* **2015**, *290*, 6168–6178. [CrossRef]
18. Ohashi, T.; Nakade, Y.; Ibusuki, M.; Kitano, R.; Yamauchi, T.; Kimoto, S.; Inoue, T.; Kobayashi, Y.; Ishii, N.; Sumida, Y.; et al. Conophylline inhibits high fat diet-induced non-alcoholic fatty liver disease in mice. *PLoS ONE* **2019**, *14*, e0210068. [CrossRef]
19. Skropeta, D.; Wei, L. Recent advances in deep-sea natural products. *Nat. Prod. Rep.* **2014**, *31*, 999–1025. [CrossRef]
20. Dumdei, E.J.; Blunt, J.W.; Munro, M.H.G.; Pannell, L.K. Isolation of Calyculins, Calyculinamides, and Swinholide H from the New Zealand Deep-Water Marine Sponge *Lamellomorpha strongylata*. *J. Org. Chem.* **1997**, *62*, 2636–2639. [CrossRef]

21. Schupp, P.J.; Kohlert-Schupp, C.; Whitefield, S.; Engemann, A.; Rohde, S.; Hemscheidt, T.; Pezzuto, J.M.; Kondratyuk, T.P.; Park, E.J.; Marler, L.; et al. Cancer chemopreventive and anticancer evaluation of extracts and fractions from marine macro- and micro-organisms collected from Twilight Zone waters around Guam. *Nat. Prod. Commun.* **2009**, *4*, 1717–1728.
22. Wright, A.D.; Schupp, P.J.; Schror, J.P.; Engemann, A.; Rohde, S.; Kelman, D.; Voogd-de, N.; Carroll, A.; Motti, C.A. Twilight zone sponges from Guam yield theonellin isocyanate and psammaplysins I and J. *J. Nat. Prod.* **2012**, *75*, 502–506. [CrossRef]
23. Wang, L.; Li, M.; Lin, Y.; Du, S.; Liu, Z.; Ju, J.; Suzuki, H.; Sawada, M.; Umezawa, K. Inhibition of cellular inflammatory mediator production and amelioration of learning deficit in flies by deep sea *Aspergillus*-derived cyclopenin. *J. Antibiot.* **2020**, *73*, 622–629. [CrossRef]
24. Bracken, A.; Pocker, A.; Raistrick, H. Studies in the biochemistry of microorganisms. Cyclopenin, a nitrogen-containing metabolic product of *Penicillium cyclopium* Westling. *Biochem. J.* **1954**, *57*, 587–595. [CrossRef]
25. Birkinshaw, J.H.; Luckner, M.; Mohammed, Y.S.; Mothes, K.; Stickings, C.E. Studies in the biochemistry of microorganisms. 114. Viridicatol and cyclopenol, metabolites of *Penicullium viridicatum* Westling and *Penicillium cyclopium* Westling. *Biochem. J.* **1963**, *89*, 196–202. [CrossRef]
26. Lu, X.; He, J.; Wu, Y.; Du, N.; Li, X.; Ju, J.; Hu, Z.; Umezawa, K.; Wang, L. Isolation and characterization of New anti-inflammatory and antioxidant components from deep marine-derived fungus *Myrothecium* sp. Bzo-1062. *Mar. Drugs* **2020**, *18*, 597. [CrossRef]
27. Yan, X.; Zhou, Y.X.; Tang, X.X.; Liu, X.X.; Yi, Z.W.; Fang, M.J.; Wu, Z.; Jiang, F.Q.; Qiu, Y.K. Macrolactins from marine-derived *Bacillus subtilis* B5 bacteria as inhibitors of inducible nitric oxide and cytokines expression. *Mar. Drugs* **2016**, *14*, 195. [CrossRef]
28. Cheng, Z.; Zhao, J.; Liu, D.; Proksch, P.; Zhao, Z.; Lin, W. Eremophilane-type Sesquiterpenoids from an *Acremonium* sp. fungus isolated from deep-sea sediments. *J. Nat. Prod.* **2016**, *79*, 1035–1047. [CrossRef]
29. Niu, S.; Liu, D.; Shao, Z.; Proksch, P.; Lin, W. Eremophilane-type sesquiterpenoids in a deep-sea fungus *Eutypella* sp. activated by chemical epigenetic manipulation. *Tetrahedron* **2018**, *74*, 7310–7325. [CrossRef]
30. Chen, S.; Wang, J.; Lin, X.; Zhao, B.; Wei, X.; Li, G.; Kaliaperumal, K.; Liao, S.; Yang, B.; Zhou, X.; et al. Chrysamides A–C, three dimeric nitrophenyl trans-epoxyamides produced by the deep-sea-derived fungus *Penicillium chrysogenum* SCSIO41001. *Org. Lett.* **2016**, *18*, 3650–3653. [CrossRef]
31. Metcalfe, D.D.; Baram, D.; Mekori, Y.A. Mast cells. *Physiol. Rev.* **1997**, *77*, 1033–1079. [CrossRef] [PubMed]
32. Kemp, S.F.; Lockey, R.F. Anaphylaxis: A review of causes and mechanisms. *J. Allergy Clin. Immunol.* **2002**, *110*, 341–348. [PubMed]
33. Noma, N.; Asagiri, M.; Takeiri, M.; Ohmae, S.; Takemoto, K.; Iwaisako, K.; Simizu, S.; Umezawa, K. Inhibition of MMP-2-mediated mast cell invasion by NF-B inhibitor DHMEQ in mast cells. *Int. Arch. Allergy Immunol.* **2015**, *166*, 84–90. [CrossRef] [PubMed]
34. Liu, Q.M.; Xie, C.L.; Gao, Y.Y.; Liu, B.; Lin, W.X.; Liu, H.; Cao, M.J.; Su, W.J.; Yang, X.W.; Liu, G.M. Deep-sea-derived butyrolactone I suppresses ovalbumin-induced anaphylaxis by regulating mast cell function in a murine model. *J. Agric. Food Chem.* **2018**, *66*, 5581–5592. [CrossRef]
35. Niu, S.; Liu, Q.; Xia, J.M.; Xie, C.L.; Luo, Z.H.; Shao, Z.; Liu, G.; Yang, X.W. Polyketides from the deep-sea-derived fungus *Graphostroma* sp. MCCC 3A00421 showed potent antifood allergic activities. *J. Agric. Food Chem.* **2018**, *66*, 1369–1376. [CrossRef]
36. Furutani, Y.; Shimada, M.; Hamada, M.; Takeuchi, T.; Umezawa, H. Reticulol, an inhibitor of cyclic nucleotide phosphodiesterases. *J. Antibiot.* **1975**, *28*, 558–560. [CrossRef]
37. Lim, D.-S.; Kwak, Y.-S.; Lee, K.-H.; Ko, S.-H.; Yoon, W.-H.; Lee, W.; Kim, C. Topoisomerase I inactivation by reticulol and its in vivo cytotoxicity against B16F10 melanoma. *Chemotherapy* **2003**, *49*, 257–263. [CrossRef]
38. Lim, D.-S.; Kwak, Y.-S.; Kim, J.-H.; Ko, S.-H.; Yoon, W.-H.; Kim, C.-H. Antitumor efficacy of reticulol from *Streptoverticillium* against the lung metastasis model B16F10 melanoma. Lung metastasis inhibition by growth inhibition of melanoma. *Chemotherapy* **2003**, *49*, 146–153. [CrossRef]
39. Hong, C.; Tontonoz, P. Liver X receptors in lipid metabolism: Opportunities for drug discovery. *Nat. Rev. Drug Discov.* **2014**, *13*, 433–444. [CrossRef]
40. El-Gendy, B.E.-D.M.; Goher, S.S.; Hegazy, L.S.; Arief, M.M.H.; Burris, T.P. Recent Advances in the Medicinal Chemistry of Liver X Receptors: Miniperspective. *J. Med. Chem.* **2018**, *61*, 10935–10956. [CrossRef]
41. Liang, X.; Zhang, X.; Lu, X.; Zheng, Z.; Ma, X.; Qi, S. Diketopiperazine-type alkaloids from a deep-sea-derived *Aspergillus puniceus* fungus and their effects on liver X receptor α. *J. Nat. Prod.* **2019**, *82*, 1558–1564. [CrossRef]
42. Gum, R.J.; Gaede, L.L.; Koterski, S.L.; Heindel, M.; Clampit, J.E.; Zinker, B.A.; Trevillyan, J.M.; Ulrich, R.G.; Jirousek, M.R.; Rondinone, C.M. Reduction of protein tyrosine phosphatase 1B increases insulin-dependent signaling in *ob/ob* mice. *Diabetes* **2003**, *52*, 21–28. [CrossRef]
43. Han, T.W.; Cai, J.; Zhong, W.; Xu, G.; Wang, F.; Tian, X.; Zhou, X.; Liu, Q.; Liu, Y.; Wang, J. Protein tyrosine phosphatase 1B (PTP1B) inhibitors from the deep-sea fungus *Penicillium chrysogenum* SCSIO 07007. *Bioorg. Chem.* **2020**. [CrossRef]
44. Koul, A.; Herget, T.; Klebl, B.; Ullrich, A. Interplay between mycobacteria and host signaling pathways. *Nat. Rev. Microbiol.* **2004**, *2*, 189–202. [CrossRef]
45. Zhou, B.; He, Y.; Zhang, X.; Xu, J.; Luo, Y.; Wang, Y.; Franzblau, S.G.; Yang, Z.; Chan, R.J.; Liu, Y.; et al. Targeting mycobacterium protein tyrosine phosphatase B for antituberculosis agents. *Proc. Natl. Acad. Sci. USA* **2010**, *107*, 4573–4578. [CrossRef]
46. Liu, Z.; Wang, Q.; Li, S.; Cui, H.; Sun, Z.; Chen, D.; Lu, Y.; Liu, H.; Zhang, W. Polypropionate derivatives with mycobacterium tuberculosis protein tyrosine phosphatase B inhibitory activities from the deep-sea-derived fungus *Aspergillus fischeri* FS452. *J. Nat. Prod.* **2019**, *82*, 3440–3449. [CrossRef]

47. Niu, S.; Si, L.; Liu, D.; Zhou, A.; Zhang, Z.; Shao, Z.; Wang, S.; Zhang, L.; Zhou, D.; Lin, W. Spiromastilactones: A new class of influenza virus inhibitors from deep-sea fungus. *Eur. J. Med. Chem.* **2016**, *108*, 229–244. [CrossRef]
48. Das, S.; Guha, I.; Chatterjee, A.; Banerji, A. Anti-cancer potential of all-*trans* retinoic acid (ATRA): A Review. *Proc. Zool. Soc.* **2013**, *66*, 1–7. [CrossRef]
49. Manasanch, E.E.; Orlowski, R.Z. Proteasome inhibitors in cancer therapy. *Nat. Rev. Clin. Oncol.* **2017**, *14*, 417–433. [CrossRef]
50. Lu, Z.; Hunter, T. Ubiquitylation and proteasomal degradation of the p21(Cip1), 27(Kip1) and p57(Kip2) CDK inhibitors. *Cell Cycle* **2010**, *9*, 2342–2352. [CrossRef]
51. Love, I.M.; Shi, D.; Grossman, S.R. p53 ubiquitination and proteasomal degradation. *Methods Mol. Biol.* **2013**, *962*, 63–73. [PubMed]
52. Feling, R.H.; Buchanan, G.O.; Mincer, T.J.; Kauffman, C.A.; Jensen, P.R.; Fenical, W. Salinosporamide A: A highly cytotoxic proteasome inhibitor from a novel microbial source, a marine bacterium of the new genus *Salinospora*. *Angew. Chem. Int. Ed.* **2003**, *42*, 355–357. [CrossRef] [PubMed]
53. Omura, S.; Fujimoto, T.; Otoguro, K.; Matsuzaki, K.; Moriguchi, R.; Tanaka, H.; Sasaki, Y. Lactacystin, a novel microbial metabolite, induces neuritogenesis of neuroblastoma cell. *J. Antibiot.* **1991**, *44*, 113–116. [CrossRef] [PubMed]
54. Groll, M.; Huber, R.; Potts, B.C.M. Crystal structures of salinosporamide A (NPI-0052) and B (NPI-0047) in complex with the 20S proteasome reveal important consequences of β-lactone ring opening and a mechanism for irreversible binding. *J. Am. Chem. Soc.* **2006**, *128*, 5136–5141. [CrossRef]
55. Ahn, K.S.; Sethi, G.; Chao, T.-H.; Neuteboom, S.T.C.; Chaturvedi, M.M.; Palladino, M.A.; Younes, A.; Aggarwal, B.B. Salinosporamide A (NPI-0052) potentiates apoptosis, suppresses osteoclastogenesis, and inhibits invasion through down-modulation of NF-κB–regulated gene products. *Blood* **2007**, *110*, 2286–2295. [CrossRef]

MDPI
St. Alban-Anlage 66
4052 Basel
Switzerland
Tel. +41 61 683 77 34
Fax +41 61 302 89 18
www.mdpi.com

Marine Drugs Editorial Office
E-mail: marinedrugs@mdpi.com
www.mdpi.com/journal/marinedrugs

www.ingramcontent.com/pod-product-compliance
Lightning Source LLC
LaVergne TN
LVHW070043120526
838202LV00101B/416